Horse and Donkey Worms and Worming

ISBN 9781451591934

Cover: Quarter Horse foal "Orphan Annie" orphaned at birth, shown at 14 weeks of age. This foal received correct worming care every 4 weeks from 4 weeks of age.

http://horsebooksandebooks.com

"Most veterinarians continue to recommend anthelmintic treatment programs for horses that are based on knowledge and concepts that are 30-40 years old."

(M.K. Nielsen, R.M. Kaplan, "Evidence-Based Equine Parasitology – It Ain't the 60s Anymore," *Proceedings des 36èmes Journées Annuelles l'Association Vétérinaire Equine Française*, 2008 - Reims, France)

"Rotation is no longer an option."

(C.R. Reinemeyer, "Controlling Strongyle Parasites of Horses: A Mandate for Change," Proceedings of the 55th Annual Convention of the American Association of Equine Practitioners, 2009.)

"The playing field has changed drastically."

(C.R. Reinemeyer, "Controlling Strongyle Parasites of Horses: A Mandate for Change," Proceedings of the 55th Annual Convention of the American Association of Equine Practitioners, 2009.)

Contents.

Introduction

In the 1960s, the dangerous worm was the large strongyle (*Strongylus vulgaris*), and worming treatment in the 1980s and 1990s targeted this worm. Today, the problem worm is the small strongyle (*cyathostome*), yet the vast majority of advice given today for worming horses is still aimed at the old regimens suited for eradicating the large strongyle (which by the way is no longer the problem). Today, the worming program should be aimed at the cyathostome – it is not the only worm of course, but it should be **the** focus of today's worming programs.

The old idea of rotation still lingers on from the early days where it was first put forward in 1966.[1] Rotation is no longer advocated by equine parasitologists.

In fact, misinformation about horse and donkey worms is all over the net, from natural therapists to, more so, chemical companies. Horses have died because of this misinformation.

It is common to find statements in advertising and about dewormers such as:
"100% effective against all worms of horses and bots."
"(*Non moxidectin, Non fenbendazole product*) safely and effectively rids horses of all major internal parasites, including tapeworms, in a single dose."
"(*Chemical*) eliminates all common horse worms and bots."
"(*Non moxidectin, Non fenbendazole product*) has the capacity to treat all common types of parasitic worms (including tapeworms) and bots."
"(*Non moxidectin, Non fenbendazole product*) has the best combined efficacy and the broadest spectrum of activity of any wormer."
"(*Product*) completely protects young horses from ascarids, as well as all other worms."

The above statements are misleading. There is no one product on the market that can be 100% effective against all worms. In fact, only moxidectin (for example, in Quest/ Equest and Farnam ComboCare) at a single dose, and fenbendazole (for example, in Panacur 100) at a double dose[2] for 5 consecutive days, are effective against some stages of encysted cyathostomes (small strongyles) – more on this later. Yet internet advertising for one product based on ivermectin even goes so far as to state, "There is no known resistance." However, resistance to ivermectin has been widely reported.[3]

Do not make the mistake of believing if something is said about a product, it must be true. I reported a false claim about dewormers to the regulatory government body in my country. I received a letter from them saying they would look into it, but over a year later, the same company is still making the same false claims.

I read an online ad for a major herbal wormer for horses which stated, "Cinnamon, for example is known for its repelling properties, especially effective against roundworm, pinworm and threadworm." However, there is no scientific evidence whatsoever to support this claim. Cinnamon has been shown to be somewhat effective against a certain parasite in the Tiger Puffer fish,[4] but that's it. Even the recent (2007) veterinary herbal medicine book, *Veterinary Herbal Medicine*, does not list deworming under the uses for cinnamon.[5]

Do not let your dogs near horse wormers, as some can cause all sorts of nasty symptoms such as pupil dilation, vomiting, convulsions, tremors, coma, respiratory failure,[6] even death.[7] If you have a dog, remove any wormer that falls on the ground after you have wormed your horse or donkey. Also, do not worm your horse near any fish ponds, as many horse wormers are also toxic to fish, turtles and tortoises. Also keep cats away from wormers.

It is also important to make sure the horse or donkey receives the full dose for its weight, as underdosing is a contributing factor to resistance. However, very special care needs to be taken to avoid overdosing donkeys and miniature equines.

On the subject of donkeys and miniature equines, these are just as susceptible as horses to worms.[8] For example, a study on 150 French donkeys found that 75.9% of them had cyathostomes.[9]

Also, some people use sheep drench for their horses in an attempt to save money – do not do this!

Signs of Worm Infestation

A horse or donkey can be looking fat, shiny and healthy and be full of worms. Never go by appearance!

The four main classes of anthelmintics used in horses and donkeys

1) Benzimidazoles
Fenbendazole
Oxibendazole
Mebendazole

2) Tetrahydropyrimidines
Pyrantel pamoate
Pyrantel tartrate

3) Macrocyclic lactones:

Avermectins
Ivermectin, abamectin, doramectin, eprinomectin, and selamectin

Milbemycins
Moxidectin and milbemycin oxime

4) Isoquinoline-pyrozines
Praziquantel

1. Large strongyles: *Strongylus vulgaris*

Ivermectin will kill both adult and immature stages of *Strongylus vulgaris*, so it's unusual to find problems with these worms anymore. This is just as well, as they like to eat away at the cecum and the colon and like to migrate and cause lots of damage[10] such as thromboembolic colic and verminous arteritis.[11] Prior to the widespread use of ivermectin, *Strongylus vulgaris* used to be a common cause of colic. They caused inflammation and architectural changes in the cranial mesenteric artery which in turn caused blockages, and this led to colic in varying degrees and sometimes to death.[12]

After the horse eats the *Strongylus vulgaris* larvae, L3s leave their previous developmental stage[13] in the small intestine, and infiltrate the mucosa (intestinal mucous membrane) and become L4s only 7 days after infection. These L4s infiltrate submucosal arteries and take off along the endothelium and reach the cecal and colic arteries 14 days after infection. Then they head off and arrive at the root of the cranial mesenteric artery 21 days after infection. After they develop for 3 to 4 months, the larvae go back to the intestinal wall via the lumen of arteries. Nodules are formed around the L5s and this happens mainly in the cecum and colon and walls. When these nodules rupture, the young adult parasites are released into the lumen of the intestine. They mature in a further 6 to 8 weeks.

Large strongyles are easy to control as they have a long Pre-Patent Period (that is, the time between infection and the first appearance of eggs) of at least 6 months, which means that once an effective wormer is given on one occasion, a whole pre-patent period needs to run its course before eggs can infect the environment.

Life Cycle of *Strongylus vulgaris*

L3 to L4 Gastrointestinal system

L4 to L5 Cranial mesenteric artery

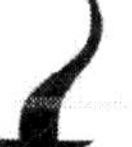

L3s eaten by horse

L5 to Adult Gastrointestinal system

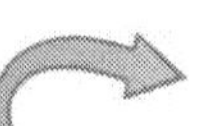

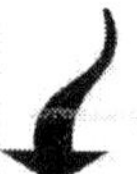

Soil and grazing L3

Eggs passed in droppings

Soil and grazing L1 to L2

2. Large strongyles: *Strongylus edentatus* and *Strongylus equinus*

The other two species of *Strongylus* in the horse are *Strongylus edentatus* and *Strongylus equinus*. Larvae of *Strongylus edentatus* enter the gut wall, go through blood vessels and head off to the liver where they stay for about 6 weeks. They leave there and turn into immature adults about 13 to 15 weeks after infection, and then they head back to the large intestine. They mature in the large intestine and the pre-patent period is approximately 11 months.[14]

Larvae of *Strongylus equinus* enter the wall of the small intestine, cecum and colon. Next they migrate to the liver where they stay for around 6 weeks, and then they head off to the pancreas on their way to the gastrointestinal tract. About 13 to 15 weeks after infection, the L5s actually penetrate the gut wall and enter the lumen of the large intestine by forming nodules.[15] The pre-patent period is approximately 9 months.

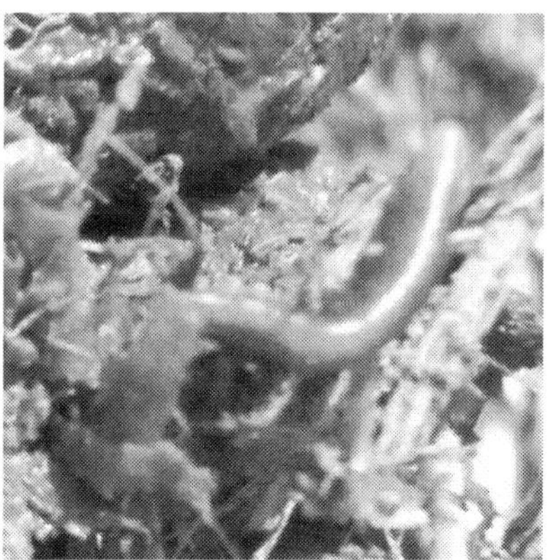

3. Roundworms (*ascarids/Parascaris equorum*)

Roundworms (*ascarids/Parascaris equorum*) can be nasty in the foal – they can migrate and cause respiratory disease, and they can also migrate to the liver just one day after being eaten by the foal. When on the ground (as opposed to in the horse) they are very, very hard to kill, even with the most determined of disinfectants, and can build up in the horse's environment and stay there for years – in paddocks, stables, anywhere the horse hangs out.[16] You could clean up manure all day long and it wouldn't make any difference with these! What makes it worse is that the females usually lay millions of eggs.[17] Bear in mind that these horrible creatures have been found in older horses too.[18]

Moxidectin (a second-generation macrocyclic lactone of the milbemycin family), ivermectin, fenbendazole, and pyrantel are effective against roundworms. Products containing these compounds all have a registered claim against adults and L4 stages, although only ivermectin has a claim for L3 stages in most European countries.

Fecal Egg Counts are too late to be of any help, as tissue inflammation will already have occurred by the time these eggs show up. However, that said, they can be of use in timing the treating. Parasitologist M.J. Murray suggests administering a dewormer when the foal is 2 months of age and then performing Fecal Egg Count 2 months later. If the eggs are still present, deworm again.[19]

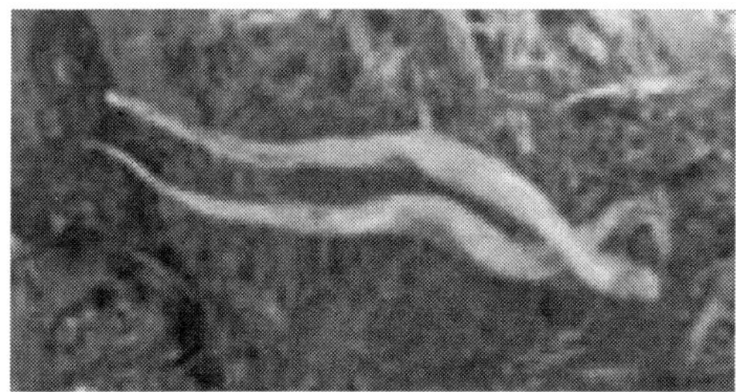

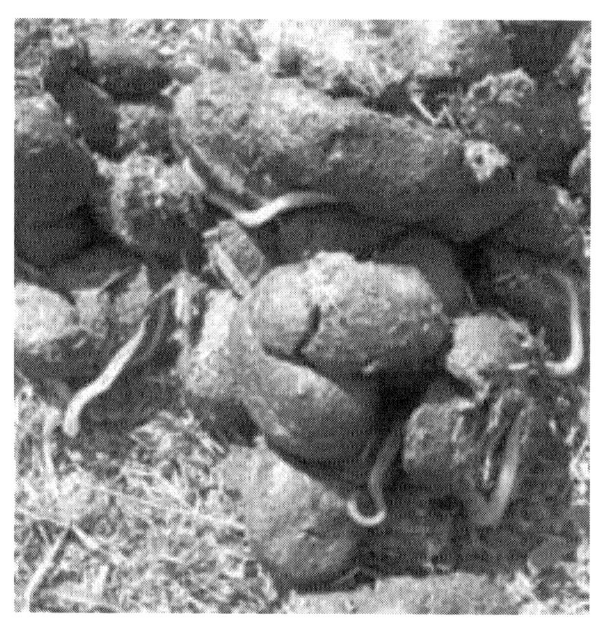

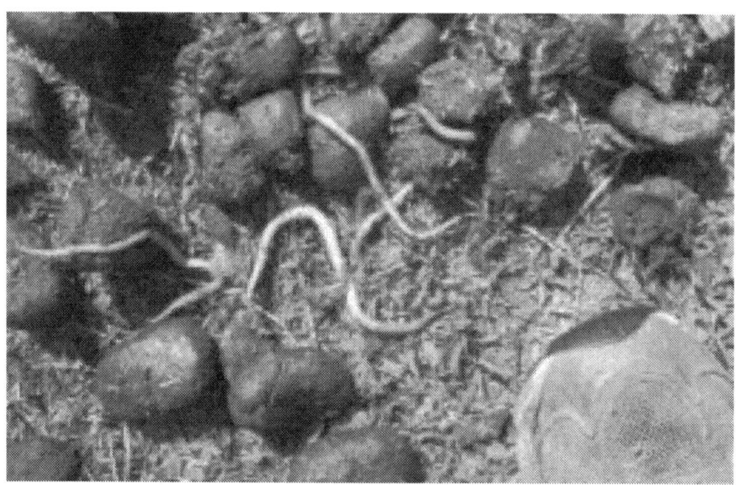

3. Bots (*Gasterophilus intestinalis*)

Bots (*Gasterophilus intestinalis*) generally aren't as nasty as the others. We have all seen bot eggs on the horse's legs and those nasty bot flies that look and sound like bees and are hard to catch! The horse eats them and they hatch in the horse's mouth, and set up residence for there for about a month. Then they turn into what is called "2nd instar larvae" and the horse swallows them. They attach to the stomach, and after having a good time in the horse for about eight to ten months, the 3rd instar larvae detach and come out in the horse's droppings. They will then pupate there and then emerge as flies three to four weeks later, and then lay eggs, and so the cycle continues.[20] The bot in the following photo was 1.2 inches (3 cm) long. A bot is the larval stage of the bot fly.

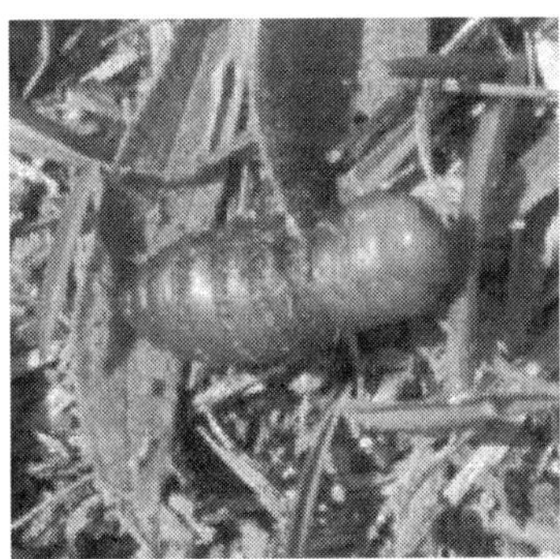

Besides the common bot, *Gasterophilus intestinalis*, there are two other species of horse bots, *Gasterophilus haemorrhoidalis*, and *Gasterophilus nasalis*. They are pretty much the same, the only difference being that *Gasterophilus intestinalis* eggs attach to the hair on the legs and shoulders, whereas the eggs of *Gasterophilus haemorrhoidalis* attach to the hairs of the lip, and the eggs of *Gasterophilus nasalis* attach to hairs under the lower jaw. The other difference is that while the 3rd instar larvae of *Gasterophilus intestinalis* and *Gasterophilus haemorrhoidalis* attach to the stomach, the 3rd instar larvae of *Gasterophilus nasalis* attach to the intestine. Bots are found all over the world. Their eggs can be removed from the legs with a bot knife (throw them out, don't let them fall on the ground!), or by scrubbing hard with warm water. The avermectin class of chemicals will dispose of them.

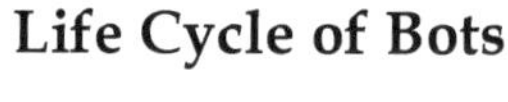

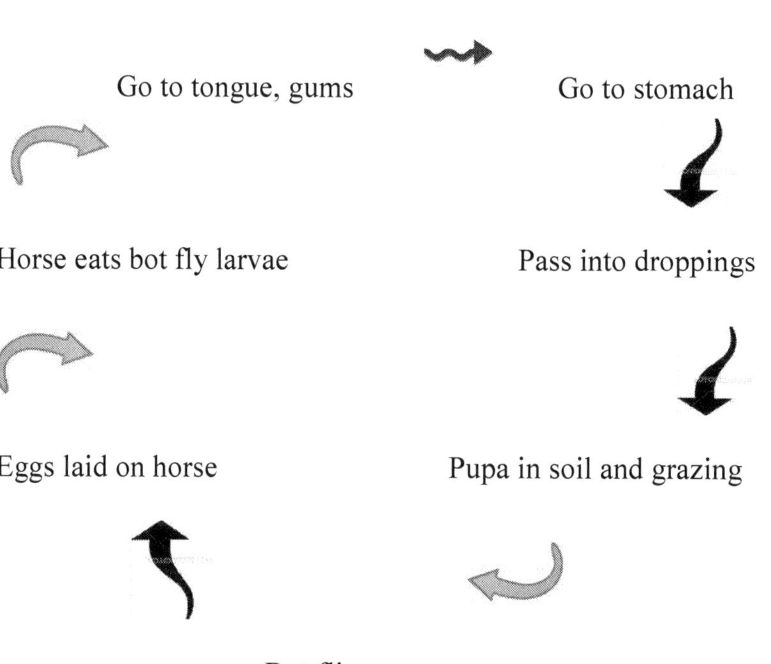

5. Small strongyles (*cyathostomes*)

Consider the life cycle of the small strongyles also called cyathostomes. The adult small strongyle lays eggs which are passed in the horse's droppings. Favorable conditions are humidity about 80%, and optimum temperature at 77ºF (25ºC). Under these conditions, the eggs passed in the manure will develop to L1 larvae within a few days.[21] With temperatures averaging 55°F (12°C), it may take weeks or months for an egg to progress to the L3 stage. No successful larvae development occurs at less than 42°F (5°C) or more than 100°F (38°C).[22] Larvae actually die at temperatures over 90°F (32°C), but can tolerate a heavy frost or freezing.[23]

The horse eats the L3 (3rd stage larvae). The L3s go into the lining of the horse's colon - *sometimes as QUICKLY as 6 HOURS* - and form a cyst. This is why they are called at that point encysted small strongyles. The wormer Equest/Quest –name depending on your country - kills many of these L3s.[24]

These are now called early L3 larvae (EL3). The EL3 larvae encyst in the mucosa or sub-mucosa of the intestine. The EL3 become hypobiotic (become inhibited L3 or IL3) and they can stay like this from anything to a few months to a few years.[25] In the northern hemisphere in northern temperate climates this happens in the winter, but in the southern temperate climates with hot summers and mild winters this happens in the summer.

75% of these L3s are actually EL3 (early 3rd stage larvae) and some are inhibited. Now, moxidectin, the chemical in Equest/Quest (different names in different countries) may not kill all EL3s in 1 dose. The registered claim of Equest/Quest and ComboCare shows that they are currently the only wormers effective as a single dose against encysted stages of small strongyles, developing stages (L), late encysted stages (LL3/EL4) and aid in control of early encysted stages (EL3) including inhibited larvae (greater than 90% effective.)[26]

Note the "aids in control." Moxidectin has not been demonstrated to be completely effective against EL3. Fenbendazole (but resistance has been demonstrated)[27] has been shown to be effective against inhibited EL3s if given for 5 consecutive days at a dose of 10 mg per 1 kg horse bodyweight[28] - this is, for example, is the recommended dose rate for Australian product Panacur 100 but in some countries such as the USA is double the recommended dose rate.

In the USA the registered claim for Panacur and Safe-Guard is, "For treatment of encysted mucosal cyathostome (small strongyle) larvae including hypobiotic early third stage, late third stage and fourth stage larvae at 10 mg/kg/day for 5 consecutive days."[29] It also states, "Fenbendazole administered orally at 10 mg/kg for 5 consecutive days to horses/ponies with naturally acquired cyathostome infection is safe and effective."

Now, NO OTHER HORSE WORMER (but moxidectin in a single dose or fenbendazole for 5 consecutive days at a certain dose rate) can affect these encysted small strongyles![30] It won't even give them a headache! You could worm your horse with standard wormers until you were blue in the face, and it would do ***nothing*** against encysted small strongyles![31]

Parasitologists Baudena, Chapman, and Horohov note that in foals previously unaffected by cyathostomes, the initial infection results in the majority of the larvae maturing to adults, whereas in adult horses which have been frequently exposed to cyathostomes, most of those worms are encysted.[32]

EL3s can stay in the horse or donkey for years,[33] or as little as 8 weeks. They eventually develop into L4 (4th stage larvae) - when this happens, they emerge from the cyst and enter the large colon (and then become L5 and adults, and the cycle starts again). If there's a huge amount of them, the emerging may kill a horse, if there are less but a lot, the horse could get colic and/or scour and /or get edema.

When they emerge they release toxins from accumulated larval waste products, and THIS is the problem with these worms.[34] Horses or donkeys can die when a huge amount of L4 burst through the colon wall and they become sick when a small number burst through.[35] This is known as "Larval Cyathostomosis."

To recap, when a horse or donkey which has a lot of encysted cyathostomes is wormed with a standard wormer, the standard wormer kills the small strongyles living in the lumen – it kills the ones of course that are not encysted. So they die and are passed out of the horse. If there were a lot of small strongyles in the lumen of the horse - guess what happens next! Because a lot of small strongyles have been killed in one go, those nasty encysted small strongyles who have been sitting safety inside the horse untouched by this standard wormer are given the signal to emerge *en masse* to replace the ones that the standard wormer killed.[36]

(If instead you worm with moxidectin (for example Equest/Quest) or a multiple-days dose of fenbendazole (for example Panacur), not only are the non-encysted adult small strongyles killed, but you will also take out a whole bunch of the encysted ones who were waiting to replace them.)

So, the standard wormer kills all the small strongyles in the lumen. The dead ones pass out of the horse in the droppings. Because they are suddenly not there anymore, the encysted small strongyles (which have been untouched and unharmed by the standard wormer) are given the signal to replace them. So a huge amount of them burst out all at once, right through the wall of the horse's large intestine.

Larval Cyathostomosis

The symptoms of Larval Cyathostomosis are weight loss, diarrhea and/or subcutaneous edema.[37] The horse may have a sudden onset of diarrhea caused by the emergence of the encysted larvae through the lining of the cecum and ventral colon. It can be life-threatening. Parasitologist Jane E. Hodgkinson states, "Furthermore, the disease is difficult to both diagnose and treat, with a high fatality rate despite intensive treatment."[38]

"The prognosis in suspected cases must be guarded because the underlying pathology can be severe without the animal showing marked clinical signs, and only less than 50% of the diarrhea cases respond to symptomatic treatment."[39]

"The disease is difficult to both diagnose and treat, with a high fatality rate despite intensive treatment."[40]

The contributing factors include seasonal conditions (autumn and winter), young horses (often 6 years of age or younger, although older horses have died from Larval Cyathostomosis), and horses recently dewormed by a wormer which cannot affect the encysted stages but which does kill the lumen-dwelling larvae and adults.[41] Parasitologist C. Monahan states, "The onset of classical larval cyathostomosis has been associated with recent anthelmintic treatments effective for removal of the lumen-dwelling stages."[42]

"The onset of classical larval cyathostomosis has been associated with recent anthelmintic treatments effective for removal of the lumen-dwelling stages."[43]

You can see the problem when there are encysted worms sitting there for possibly 3 years, worms that your standard wormer won't touch, so someone could be worming the horse religiously with standard wormers and the encysted worms won't be affected in the slightest.

Research has shown that cyathostomes have become more and more important as a cause of sickness and death in horses, and today are considered the main reason for worming horses.[44]

A standard wormer - other than a single dose of Equest/Quest or ComboCare or a 5 day dose of Fenbendazole/Panacur - does NOTHING against encysted small strongyles, it has NO EFFECT whatsoever.

If you have never given moxidectin (- or fenbendazole for 5 consecutive days at the recommended dose for encysted small strongyles -) well.... that could be a cause for concern, depending on your geographical location, and your horse's circumstances. Of course, some horses are more prone to worm infestation than others – the old saying "Some of the horses have most of the worms" is correct. Many healthy horses have an effective immune response to worms which keeps the numbers low, unless the horse becomes sick, badly fed or gets a large number of worms. Parasitologists consider that in any group of horses, 20% will carry 80% of the worm burden.[45] This, by the way, may lead to natural alleged dewormers wrongfully getting the credit for being successful.[46]

At any rate, egg counts do not show how badly a horse is infested with encysted small strongyles. This means the egg count could be zero but the horse could be infested with these worms.

I'll repeat this! Egg counts do NOT show how badly a horse is infested with encysted small strongyles. This means the egg count could be ZERO but the horse could be INFESTED with these worms.

What even many veterinary surgeons do not say on their websites is that the only active ingredient that kills encysted small strongyles in a single dose is moxidectin, available in, for example, Equest/Quest (name depending on which country you live in) or ComboCare. Fenbendazole at the dose rate of 10 mg/kg over a 5 day course is also effective.

I recently saw a popular wormer brochure that stated, "100% effective" and the same claim was made on the company's website. This is a false claim, as those wormers were not fenbendazole or moxidectin, so could not be 100% effective. In fact, no wormer can claim to be 100% effective, but the chemicals in the advertised wormers had no registered claim to affect encysted small strongyles. How did the company get away with these false claims? I have no idea, but the point is, they did! In fact at the time of writing, these claims are still on their advertising material and on their websites.

As just mentioned, fenbendazole, the active ingredient in, for example, Panacur, can kill some of the encysted stages including L3 if given 5 days in a row at 10 mg per kg.[47] Resistance to a single dose of fenbendazole for encysted cyathostomes has been demonstrated,[48] you do need to give it for 5 consecutive days.

Fenbendazole (Panacur) effectively treats and controls large strongyles (adults and migrating larval stages of *Strongylus vulgaris*; adults and tissue larval stages of *Strongylus edentatus*), small strongyles (cyathostomes) including encysted early 3rd stage (hypobiotic), late third stage and fourth stage mucosal cyathostome larvae, pinworms (*Oxyuris equi*), ascarids (*Parascaris equorum*), and arteritis (inflammation of the walls of the arteries) caused by 4th stage larvae of *Strongylus vulgaris* in horses.[49]

Parasitologists Swiderski and French state that dosing with fenbendazole may be inferior to moxidectin in the prevention of the introduction of resistant worms in new arrivals and suggest that new arrivals should be treated with fenbendazole regimens followed by a single dose administration of a macrocyclic lactone to remove the remaining worms.[50] This is the regime I personally use.

A horse can be fat and shiny and have a heavy worm infestation. Fat shiny horses have died from worms. Don't be fooled into thinking a horse is not heavily infested with worms just by appearance.

If you have read my book *Natural Horse Care The Right Way*, you will know that I have often spoken with Maria Daraio of Dara Park Stud in Australia about the tragedy of thinking that natural wormers and certain chemical wormers are efficient. Both Maria and I have seen horses die horrible deaths from encysted cyathostomes. Maria's story is in that book, but it is so important that I have repeated it here. Maria breeds Arabians as well as Quarter Horses. I asked Maria to write about her experiences with Larval Cyathostomosis, and this is what she said:

Our problem with cyathostomes began in 2001 when a rising yearling Quarter Horse filly suddenly started to scour seriously. She went from a nice, round filly in excellent condition, to a rake in a matter of days and we called the vet in to deal with it. We had no idea what was wrong with her and we fought for weeks to pull her through.

She was put onto drips, antibiotics by the bucketloads and I remember using our big tree to hitch up the drip in the dark. She suffered greatly and was humanely euthanized not long after she developed a neck abscess due to having so many injections. The vets were absolutely in the dark as to what had caused it.

For the next five years we embarked on a horrible rollercoaster ride whereby we periodically would see an otherwise healthy youngster come down with serious scours, get treated by one vet or other and then ultimately die. Not all died and we did experience varying degrees of success in saving these sick horses. Each time the nightmare would repeat itself and we began to notice a correlation between the onset of the scouring and the onset of wet, cold weather. We mentioned this to our then vet and he just shrugged his shoulders and continued to prescribe one antibiotic or other.

We also then went through a stage where new born foals were coming down with deadly scours at anything from a week to twenty-eight days after birth. Again they were plied with all the top shelf antibiotics available under veterinary supervision.

Some foals survived whilst others did not. We soon discovered that the white anti-scour powder that the vets were invariably supplying was absolutely useless, and that any foal injected with just procaine penicillin was also doomed to die.

The vets at this stage decided that these foals were suffering from salmonella even though the bug itself was only ever found in ONE horse. (Not surprising since our research suggested that all horses carry the bug. It is under duress that it proliferates and then causes problems). The vets stopped looking for a cause after this as they believed they'd found the cause in Salmonella.

I was even chastised when I decided to treat one of our sick youngsters myself as I was pregnant at the time. The vet felt it was too dangerous for me and my unborn child since the filly was carrying a deadly bacteria. Unfortunately, unless I wanted her to die, I had no choice but to medicate her.

Time wore on and every season we'd lose both foals and older youngsters to the mysterious 'bug'. Those that survived ended up looking shocking and never thrived. It was a chance visit to another stud that saw the introduction of 'Protexin' to the recovery regime. From then on, at least the survivors would actually recover with no apparent side effects. Then the season we bred our A class supreme champion filly, Dara Park Sarina, we had a good 75% of our foal crop come down with the 'scouring bug' and we nearly lost Sarina. (Photo following).

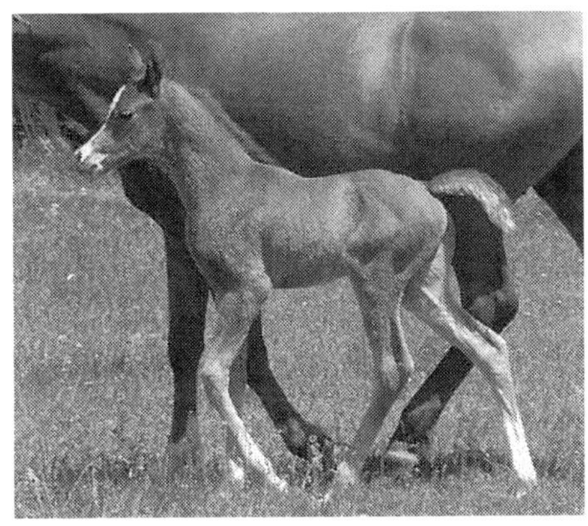

She was born an absolutely stunning filly and we knew she was special. But within the eight days of life she came down with the scouring. We were desperate to save her. The vet we were using by this stage was in my opinion arrogant enough to think he was better than any of the other vets and that he knew what the problem was. He insisted it was clostridia and the fact that our property had been a cattle farm before we bought it sealed it for him. He supplied us with a new antibiotic and advised us to use Scourban. The filly kept deteriorating and it was obvious we were going to lose her. I called another vet and she prescribed throwing out the antibiotic and putting her onto Protexin instead. I'd seen too many foals die of this problem and I was not interested in allowing this filly to die so I refused to do so. What I did do was to combine the two treatments as well as adding Gastroshield to the mix. Unbelievably, the next morning, instead of waking to a dead filly foal, I found her very much on the road to recovery!

Whilst we'd stumbled onto the correct treatment of the symptoms, we were still none-the-wiser as to what was actually causing the problem. By this stage the 'bug' had moved onto our gorgeous black Arabian pony mare, Gembrook Halloween. We fought for several months to save her with all sorts of things tried. Unfortunately she was in foal and this limited what could be administered. She foaled early and seemed to recover suddenly. But then at two days post foaling disaster struck and the mare collapsed. The foal was under her and when she went to get back up again she stepped on the filly's leg and snapped it in half. To cut a long story short, we saved that filly but lost the mare two months later. It had been a four month battle which we unfortunately lost due to vets being caught unaware. Halley had stopped scouring but had become severely anemic and lactating was just too much for her. Whilst they worked hard to save the filly with regular changes of casts and x-rays to her leg, it had never crossed their minds to check the mare's blood levels.

Then a breakthrough occurred! A two year old Quarter Horse colt became sick and then started to scour badly. By this stage our vet clinic had two new young vets who were not so convinced they knew the answers. They fought long and hard to save Player but unfortunately we lost him one cold night. The vets came out and by the lights of their car they did an autopsy, taking every organ that they could. They were adamant they were going to find out the answer to what was causing the problem and find out they did. I can still remember the wording of the autopsy report. There was no evidence of anything wrong with the colt! All they could find was 'an unusually large load of cyathostomes'. So there it was.........WORMS!

We had always employed a strong worming program and whenever the vets came to see yet another sick horse, they would always ask, 'Has this horse been wormed?' Our answer was always 'Yes!' They never once asked had we wormed the horse with Equest. That one question would have saved so many horses and it really makes us angry to consider this. We felt betrayed as we'd always looked after our horses very well and had always drenched regularly. Player had gone from a healthy 2 y.o. to very sick very quickly. We originally did a fecal worm count as soon as he became sick. It showed a ZERO worm count!!!! We were informed after the autopsy results came through that encysted cyathostome eggs do not show up in a fecal worm count as encysted cyathostomes do not lay eggs. The entire herd of horses at Dara Park was ordered to be drenched with Equest THREE times over SIX WEEKS.

It took another couple of years to learn about looking after our dung beetles and about harrowing in the middle of summer to kill the worm larvae. Once this was all in place, we had no further problems with scouring horses. These days we make sure the horses get a dose of Equest in January as it is the ONLY wormer that kills the cyathostomes in a single dose when they are actually encysted within the horse's gut. Then they get done again once the weather changes from Summer to the first Autumn rains. Throughout the wet times of the year we dose them with Equest. Every broodmare is drenched the day she foals with Equest and then the foals are drenched with another dung beetle friendly drench as of one month of age. Then they get their first Equest dose at three months of age.

Since adopting the above regime, we have not had to open the Scourban bottle and although we always have the appropriate antibiotics, probiotics and Gastroshield in the fridge, we have not had occasion to use it. It has been a long journey and I shake my head in disbelief when I read the comments from some ill-informed horse owners who think that following the 'natural' worming approaches are going to protect their horses. Every time I read about some poor horse suddenly becoming sick and passing away in agony, I grit my teeth as I know how hopelessly ill-equipped to handle this problem most vets actually are. Too many of them are completely ignorant of the vital importance of including Equest in one's worming regime for one's horses. Too many are ignorant of how to actually save a horse that comes down with a proliferation of the worm. Too many owners are also in the dark when it comes to encysted cyathostomes.

When a horse is not treated as outlined above, the cyathostomes burrow into the horse's gut. Once here they are completely immune to any of the other otherwise efficient wormers. This happens over the Summer months here. Once the weather starts to change and it gets wet, these worms migrate from the gut wall and leave sometimes a heavily damaged gut behind. This damaged gut becomes infected and inflamed which is why the horse now needs antibiotics. Unfortunately, if the inflammation is too severe, the horse now also needs steroid treatment to help arrest the severe scouring as well as the Scourban. The treatment now appears simple enough but this is certainly one case where prevention is far better than cure. A great deal of suffering on the part of the horse can be avoided if it is placed on a worming program that includes Equest.

The above heartbreaking story about her experience with Larval Cyathostomosis was written by Maria Daraio of Dara Park Stud in Australia. Her website is http://www.darapark.net

In many cases, horses may show no signs of encysted small strongyles at all and appear perfectly healthy for some time. Encysted small strongyles can sit in the lining of the colon for 2 to

3 years or more and there is no way to detect their presence, no way at all. Many sudden mysterious deaths usually attributed by default to snakebite actually may well be due to Larval Cyathostomosis. I have known of horses who were fine and fat and shiny in the morning to be dead suddenly that night from Larval Cyathostomosis. In fact, I knew of two in 2008 who were from a hot dry climate out in western NSW, Australia.

6. Tapeworms

Tapeworms have been associated with colic,[51] specifically spasmodic colic (22%), impaction colic (81%) and 100% of intussusception colic.[52] The colic often recurs and the site where the tapeworms were attached often becomes infected or abscessed.[53]

There are three species of equine tapeworms: *Anoplocephala perfoliata*, *Anoplocephaloides mamillana*, and *Anoplocephala magna*.

The occurrence of tapeworms varies by location, but far more horses in temperate climates are affected.[54] There does not appear to be an acquired or age resistance to this parasite in horses because all ages, including older ones, can be infected.[55]

A horse needs to eat mites containing the cysticercoid stage of the parasite to become infected with a tapeworm. These mites are normal soil mites which live in pasture, in hay, and even in processed feedstuffs.

Tapeworm segments[56] contain both male and female organs. As they develop, their eggs disintegrate in the large intestine, and are passed in the manure. The mites eat the tapeworm eggs, which develop for 2 to 4 months inside the mite before reaching the infective stage.[57]

Fecal Egg Counts are of little use in detecting tapeworm infestation. Murray noted, "In one report, fecal examinations were negative for tapeworm eggs unless there were at least 40 tapeworms in the horse."[58]

For several years, pyrantel products have been used at a double dose to treat for tapeworms in horses. Murray notes that praziquantel is effective in killing tapeworms at dosages ranging from 1.0 mg/kg to 2.5 mg/kg[59] and the *Merck Veterinary Manual* states that praziquantel (at 1 mg/kg) appears to be effective in removing *Anoplocephaloides mamillana* but that pyrantel products are not.[60] However, Murray states that normal dosages (6.6 mg/kg) of pyrantel pamoate are 87% effective, while double the normal dosage is greater than 93% effective.[61] Murray also notes that pyrantel tartrate (2.65 mg/kg) removes *Anoplocephala* species.[62] Reinemeyer *et.al.* noted that in two dose-confirmation studies, a single oral treatment of pyrantel pamoate at a dose rate of 13.2 mg/kg was greater than 95.5% effective against *Anoplocephala perfoliata* in naturally-infected horses.[63]

Murray notes that the traditional recommendation to treat in the spring and the fall, has not been critically examined and that exposure to mites may occur at other times of the year.[64]

7. Lungworms (Dictyocaulus arnfieldi)

Donkeys are generally named as the culprit in carrying these worms and infecting horses. However, lungworms have been found in horses with no previous donkey contact[65] and transmission from horse to horse has been discovered.[66] With horses, it used to be considered that lungworms are usually only of concern in foals, but infections have been found in horses up to 20 years of age, and it is now considered that horses do not have age immunity to lungworms.[67] However, foals are far more susceptible than adult horses.[68]

Mature lungworms live in the bronchioles and grow up to just over 3 inches (8 cm) long. They lay eggs in the air ways. The donkeys or horses cough up the eggs, then swallow them, and the eggs hatch along their way to being passed out in the manure.[69] The infective stage only takes five days on pasture. After they are swallowed, the infective larvae migrate from the intestine via the lymphatics and the pulmonary arterial system to the bronchioles and bronchi where they mature. Lungworm larvae do not generally develop into adults in the mature horse.

Horses and donkeys infected with lungworms can have a persistent dry cough. It has been reported that the response to lungworm in horse varies greatly with the individual.[70] Research has found however that there is no seasonal variation in lungworm and that adult lungworms have been found in the lungs of horses and donkeys throughout the year.[71]

Generally, donkeys will not present with any clinical signs despite having large lungworm burdens.[72] However, secondary problems related to lungworm infestation include influenza.[73]

These are difficult to detect in the live horse, and the usual diagnosis is the discovery of eosinophills in tracheal mucus.[74]

However, they can be detected in the live donkey by the modified Baermann technique of Fecal Egg Count, if appropriate care is taken with the samples.[75]

Thiabendazole at the dose rate of 440 mg/kg has also been used successfully to treat donkeys and horses.[76] However, some horses and donkeys showed depression and anorexia after treatment.[77] Another study used oxibendazole at the dose rate of 5 to 15 mg/kg, and found it to be ineffective against lungworm.[78] Likewise, a single dose of fenbendazole at the dose rate of 7.5 mg/kg to 30 mg/kg) and repeated treatments (2 x 15 mg/kg) also failed to eliminate lungworm infections in donkeys.[79] In one trial in donkeys, mebendazole was ineffective when given orally at a dose rate of 4.3 to 5.7 mg/kg for five days but when given at the higher dose rates of 15.2 to 20 mg/kg was 75 to 100% effective.[80]

An older study recommended that in a situation of donkey-only grazing, donkeys can be treated for lungworm in the spring, and new arrivals should be isolated and treated.[81] A more recent study found that donkeys treated with moxidectin tested negative for lungworm larvae 21 days after treatment.[82] Other studies have shown that ivermectin in combination with change to non contaminated pasture was effective.[83] Albendazole (Valbazen) at the dose rate of 25 mg/kg twice daily for five days has been demonstrated to eliminate lungworm infections in horses.[84] Thiemann and Bell state that treatment of choice in donkeys is ivermectin at 200 mg/kg.[85] They also state that reinfestation is slow, especially if ivermectin or moxidectin is being used.[86] The Merck Veterinary Manual also recommends ivermectin or moxidectin for lungworm treatment.[87] Purdy suggests treatment for lungworms in horses and donkeys is ivermectin with a repeat treatment in three weeks.[88]

Lungworm larvae can live for a long time in a cool, moist environment, but will not survive a heavy frost.

8. Pinworms (Oxyuris equi)

These worms are not particularly important. They are the cause of the horse rubbing its tail. This only happens when the worms emerge to lay their eggs. If your horse rubs its tail, wash the area with warm water to clean off the worms and then dispose of the cloth or towel immediately. The eggs will fall off the horse and cling to fences, feed bins, buckets, or anything else in the environment, and infect other horses.

Pinworms do not do much damage to the horse, and ivermectins kill them easily. The adults live mainly in the small colon. The female is 3 to 6 inches (7.5 to 15 cm) long and the males are much smaller, and there are fewer males about. The eggs show up in a routine Fecal Egg Count.

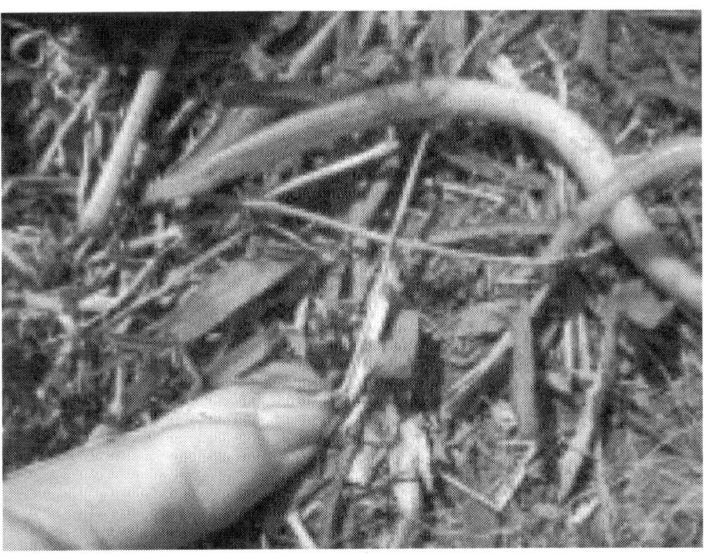

9. Stomach worm (*Trichostrongylus axei*)

The mature stomach worm lives, as you would expect, in the stomach. This worm if present in large numbers has been known to cause mild intestinal disturbances and chronic catarrhal gastritis. The adults penetrate the mucosa and produce nodular areas resulting in thickened mucosa causing erosions and ulcerations.[89] The horse eats the 3rd stage infective larvae from hatched eggs on the ground, the manure comes out with eggs in it, and the horse eats these eggs, quite direct. Other fun facts about this worm are that it is small, less than 1/3rd inch long (8 mm) and also infects ruminants.

10. Warbles

Warbles are the larvae of the bovine (cattle) warble flies (*Hypoderma bovis* and *Hypoderma lineatum*). These are quite uncommon in horses. They are a cattle worm, but as ivermectin kills them easily it's pretty rare to find them in either horses or cattle these days. At any rate, they are usually found only in horses which are kept near cattle.

The adult flies attach their eggs to the hair on the lower legs. The eggs hatch and the larvae penetrate the skin, migrate, and end up at the neck, back or withers where they form nodules. The larvae usually die in the horse, but in cattle they mature and emerge through the skin.

11. Threadworm (Strongyloides westeri)

Threadworm usually affects foals under 6 months of age[90] where it lives in the small intestine. However, mares sometimes harbor larval stages which are activated by foaling which causes them to move to the udder where the worm is transmitted via the milk to the foal.[91] Ivermectin has a registered claim to kill them[92] as does oxibendazole.[93]

12. Liver fluke (*Fasciola hepatica*)

The horse is not a natural host for the liver fluke, and again, Fecal Egg Counts are of no use detecting this worm. Signs of infestation in the horse are irregular heartbeat, weight loss, and chronically soft manure.

Damage to the liver is caused by the migration of the immature fluke. Adult fluke live (and lay eggs) in the bile ducts where they drink blood and cause tissue irritation. These eggs hatch into an immature fluke ("miracidium"), which then infiltrates a snail in a wet or damp area. The fluke egg needs to fall into water for the miracidium to develop. In the summer, this takes two to four weeks at summer temperatures. The infectious stage becomes encysted on grass, and the fluke is eaten by the horse or donkey.

One study found that a patent infection was established in only one out of ten horses given oral doses of up to 800 metacercariae[94] (encased encysted stage) and concluded, "The experimental data show that the horse exhibits a pronounced resistance to the establishment of a liver fluke infection."[95] These findings were in agreement with an earlier South African study.[96] However, a Bolivian study in a high endemic region for *Fasciola hepatica* found that donkeys are a main host in that region.[97]

One study asserted that a safe method of treatment for infected horses is an oral dose of oxyclozanide at a dose rate of 15 ml/50 kg body weight.[98]

13. Chemical dewormers

Safety of chemical wormers

Sadly, there is a lot of unfounded nonsense around about the supposed dangers of chemical wormers. Here are the facts. Herbal wormers do NOT work against the deadlier varieties of horse worms, and these worms do KILL horses. We do need to use chemical wormers, very sad but also very true.

Now, these days, chemical wormers made for horses are very safe.[99] Some wormers are safer than others. You will see unsupported false scaremongering on the net that Equest/Quest (moxidectin) is unsafe in a small overdose. In the USA, Quest is registered for foals over the age of 6 months. It used to be 4 months of age, but misuse of the product in dogs caused the age downgrade.[100] In Australia, Equest (same product, different name) is recommended for foals over the age of 2 months.

At any rate, you must be careful not to overdose Quest/Equest in foals. You can ask your veterinary surgeon to come and estimate your foal's weight, or you can go to this website (http://www.gaitedhorses.net/Articles/horseweight.html) where you can enter the girth and length, and the site calculates the estimated weight. Be VERY careful with weight tapes as they can be inaccurate.

A Drug Tolerance Test on Quest[101] (also known as "Equest," and the active ingredient being moxidectin) –administered five times, and six times the recommended dose rate of Quest Plus Gel to young foals and horses. Fourteen hours after treatment, one foal given five times the recommended dose rate showed ataxia, incoordination, lethargy, depression, and droopy lips and eyelids. This foal was stated to be "normal" by the 24 hour observation point. Another foal also showed ataxia, incoordination, lethargy, depression and droopy lips and eyelids at 24 hours post treatment, and this foal returned to normal by the 48 hour observation point.

It also noted that two of the four foals that received a dose at five times the recommended dose rate did not show any signs of adverse reaction.

The study stated, "All animals returned to normal by 48 hours post treatment."

One of the two yearlings administered Quest Plus Gel at five times the recommended dose showed ataxia, incoordination, lethargy, depression, and droopy lips and eyelids at 23 hours post treatment and returned to normal by the 48 hour observation point. Both yearlings that were administered Quest Plus Gel at six times the recommended dose also showed ataxia, incoordination, lethargy, depression and droopy lips and eyelids at 14 hours post treatment. Both yearlings had returned to normal by the 24 hour observation point.[102]

The trial Target Animal Toxicity Study – Study No. 0696-E-US-08-01 did extensive tests on four month old foals, some on 4 times the recommended dose level of Quest weekly for three weeks. Hematology, Coagulation, Serum Chemistry, and Urinalysis were carried out on the foals and the results stated, "A comparison of pre and post treatment hematology, coagulation, clinical chemistry, and urinalysis values indicated no biologically significant changes." Pathology observations were as follows, "No gross lesions suggestive of treatment-related toxicity were observed at necropsy. Similarly, microscopic evaluation of all major tissues obtained from test animals in the high-dose (4X) group at necropsy revealed no histopathologic changes indicative of a toxic effect."

The conclusion of Target Animal Toxicity Study – Study No. 0696-E-US-08- 01 was as follows, "Under the conditions of this study, 12 of the foals treated with the final Quest Plus Gel formulation showed transient signs including slight depression, slight ataxia, and/or droopy lips. All affected test foals returned to normal without intervention or significant long-term health effects. No other clinical or pathological effects were noted in any of the treated foals."

Don't overdo chemical wormers!

Equest/Quest (moxidectin) does not need to be given as regularly as other wormers (as it has been demonstrated to have an 84 day Egg Reappearance Period[103] as opposed to 56 days for ivermectin[104]), so use it according to instructions. This reduces the amount of chemical wormer going into your horse.

Q: What happens to the encysted cyathostomes killed by moxidectin or fenbendazole?

A: They simply dissolve and are reabsorbed.

14. Herbal and "natural" dewormers - not for horses!

Black walnut. Has been shown to cause severe laminitis, and has been used by veterinary researchers specifically to bring on laminitis.[105]

Wormwood. The main variety is *Artemisia absinthium* and this is what absinthe is made from. Wormwood contains the toxic chemical *monoterpene thujone* and this is why many countries have banned the use and production of absinthe. It is a neurotoxin and has been shown to cause brain damage.[106] It traditionally was used to control roundworms in people, which is how it got its common name, "wormwood." Long term use in people has been shown to cause hallucinations, tremors, convulsions, and even paralysis.[107]

However, a recent study concluded, "The results of the present study suggest that A. absinthium extracts are a promising alternative to the commercially available anthelmintics for the treatment of GI nematodes of sheep."[108]

Purgatives: Cascara, senna, aloe
These are used as laxatives and the aim in using them for worm control is to cause bowel contractions in order to expel worms. Of course, this requires that worms are in the bowel in the first place, and it doesn't take much common sense to see why it's not a good idea to induce scouring in a horse!

Garlic as a wormer
There is zero evidence for this, and anyway, you should not feed garlic to your horse due to the reported toxicities[109] and risk of Heinz Body Anaemia.
There is no scientific evidence that garlic is helpful for horses, rather, there is scientific evidence from several scientific studies that garlic is harmful to horses.[110] The feeding of garlic has been shown to cause Heinz body anemia.[111] It has been demonstrated that chronic supplementation with garlic at certain levels, beginning

with less than 0.2 g/kg per day (100 grams = 3 ½ ounces in 1,100 lb = 500 kg horse) resulted in Heinz body anemia, as characterized by reduced red blood cell count, free hemoglobin, hematocrit, and haptoglobin; increased free bilirubin, mean red cell hemoglobin, mean red cell volume, platelets and incidence of Heinz bodies.[112]

One study found that the risk of feeding freeze dried garlic begins at 100 grams (3.5 ounces) per day.[113] Another study, by W. Pearson, has been cited on the net along with several inaccuracies.

Let's get this out of the way first. W. Pearson states, "However, natural is not synonymous with safe, and horses will voluntarily consume enough garlic to cause Heinz body anemia which, if left unchecked, can be fatal."[114] Pearson has now agreed that the horses in the study ate the large quantities of garlic due to the fact it was fed with molasses.[115] Now to the inaccuracies.

Inaccuracy 1
"She (Pearson) found that the garlic eaters showed changes in their blood chemistry beginning at around the third week, when garlic intake was four cups (560 grams) of freeze dried garlic per day."[116]
Facts
Incorrect. Toxicity in the trial began at less than 0.2 g/kg per day, that's 100 grams (3 ½ ounces) for a 500 kg (approx. 1,100 lb) horse, not 560 grams – 100 grams is a lot less than 560 grams!
A cup is a measure of volume, not weight. W. Pearson of course did not mention "cups" as it was a scientific study. However, if 1 cup of freeze dried garlic does weigh 140 grams, then almost ¾ of a cup of freeze dried garlic fed to horse per day is a toxic level!

W. Pearson wrote to me, "We need a lot more research before we can argue strongly either for or against its longterm use in horses."[117] The reason for this is, that they do not know if the anemia which showed up in the third week of Pearson's trial (as stated above) was caused by an increase in the dose of the garlic, or by the length of time the horses had been consuming the garlic. Her trial was a volumetric analysis (titrating) trial, starting with a total daily dose of 0.1 g/kg/day, working up to 0.5 g/kg/day over a six week period.

However, as I have said, the study found that garlic was toxic to horses in an amount as small as 100 grams (3 ½ ounces) a day.[118] Why would you want to feed your horse garlic? If your horse is about to be attacked by vampires, then it's a good idea. Otherwise, bear in mind there is no evidence that garlic has any benefits at all for horses, and much evidence to show it is unsafe. Many people feed garlic, and as their horses do not die or become ill, and even look well, they assume garlic must be safe. If you want your horses to be the healthiest they can be, don't assume that they are healthy just because they aren't showing any obvious symptoms yet. There is a wide area between looking sickly and optimum health!

Garlic has been shown to be beneficial in some other animals. Don't forget, what's good for one animal is not always good for another. Lots of us eat chocolate, but it is commonly fatal to dogs. Garlic has been shown to lower cholesterol and triglyceride levels in humans, dogs and monkeys.[119] A study on the effect of garlic on blood pressure in human patients with and without elevated systolic blood pressure found that garlic did reduce systolic blood pressure in those patients who did have elevated systolic blood pressure.[120] Another study focused on a certain odorless form of garlic rich in bioavailable water-soluble organosulfur compound, which had a higher antioxidant activity than fresh garlic and none of its adverse effects. It concluded that the available evidence suggests that garlic in this form was of potential benefit in humans in reducing risk factors for cardiovascular and cerebrovascular diseases and dementia, including Alzheimer's disease.[121]

Yet there is no evidence that garlic is safe for horses. Noted equine nutritionist and vet Dr Eleanor Kellon advises not to feed it.[122]

Claim

This is not to do with worms but is worth mentioning. Another claim which has been made in support of feeding garlic to horses, is that it is effective against the bacteria Heliobacter pylori and thus may be helpful against ulcers in horses. (Heliobacter pylori is a factor in human ulcers.)

Fact

Heliobacter pylori has not been found in horses.[123]

Sage

Apart from the fact there is not a drop of evidence to suggest sage as a wormer for horses, sage has been shown to cause photosensitivity in sheep.[124]

Tansy

All species of tansy are toxic.[125] The common tansy used for horses also contains the neurotoxin thujone. The FDA does not allow the oral use of tansy in humans, only in the case of alcoholic beverages which must first be shown to be thujone free.[126]

Rue

This is a wonderful herb with lots of excellent properties. It has been named to have an anthelmintic (getting rid of worms) effect in other species, although no studies have as yet shown it can dispose of horse worms.

Pumpkin seeds

In 1918, researchers found pumpkin seeds were efficient in killing earthworms.[127] Pumpkin seeds have been used as dewormers for roundworms and tapeworms in people, but this is to be followed by a salt water purge then a castor oil purge.[128]

Chamomile

No evidence as a wormer for horses, however is a most beneficial herb.

Thyme

Traditionally used to kill intestinal worms in humans. Trials have shown that the use of certain herbs including thyme can prevent large round worm (*Ascaris suum*) infections in pigs. The trials found that a mixture of thyme, lemon balm and purple coneflower in the feed of pigs resulted in a significant prevention against round worms. As the high dosage needed to be effective was not economically feasible, they investigated whether they could lower the dosage, and whether the addition of black tea would help the herb mixture. They did this on the grounds that black tea is rich in tannins. Tannins are said to limit the amount of worm eggs produced, and the black tea interferes with the worms attaching to the intestinal mucosal layer.[129]

The study concluded, "A diet with a herb mixture containing 1% Thymus vulgaris, 1% Melissa officinalis and 1% Echinacea purpurea for growing and finishing pigs does not decrease the number of pigs which are infected with Ascaris suum, but does reduce the average number of worms in the gastro intestinal tract. The addition of 1% black tea to this herb mixture does not result in a lower number of infected pigs and also does not reduce the average number of worms in pigs."[130]

The study suggested that, "On organic farms with a low worm infection rate, probably a combination of conventional synthetic drugs and a diet with herb mixture containing 1% Thymus vulgaris, 1% Melissa officinalis and 1% Echinacea purpurea is an option."[131]

Yarrow (*Achillea millefolium*)

A 2008 study concluded that, "the entire plant of A. millifolium possesses significant anthelmintic activity and could be a potential alternative for treating cases of helminth infections in ruminants."[132] (Don't forget, a horse is not a ruminant!)

Ginger

A recent study on ginger concluded, "This study shows that ginger possesses in vivo anthelmintic activity in sheep thus justifying the age-old traditional use of this plant in helminth infestation."[133]

Iris hookeriana

A 2008 study concluded that, "From the present study it can be suggested that *I. hookeriana* rhizome exhibited significant anthelmintic activity against gastrointestinal nematodes of sheep and has the potential to contribute to the control of gastrointestinal nematode parasites of small ruminants."[134]

Others

A recent study showed that herbal wormer using Artemisia vulgaris (mugwort), Foeniculum vulgare (fennel), and Hyssopus officinalis had no effectiveness in goats against Gastrointestinal nematodes, which the paper said are the most important worms in ruminants.[135] A study by some of the same researchers found that garlic failed to control gastrointestinal nematodes in goats and papaya seeds failed to control gastrointestinal nematodes in lambs.[136] However, another study showed that papaya seed was effective against the parasites *Aspiculuris tetraptera* and *Hymenolepis nana* in mice.[137]

The papaya tree latex anthelmintic against gastrointestinal nematodes of monogastric animals has been researched widely and shown to be effective against worms in some species.[138] Papaya latex was effective against ascarids in chicken[139] and pigs,[140] but another study suggested that Papaya latex was less effective against *Haemochus contortus* in sheep.[141] Results of previous trials suggest that the latex has a high safety margin when given to poultry.[142] However, it caused high toxicity when given to ruminants and a high dose was shown to produce either mild diarrhoea or constipation in pigs[143] and mice.[144]

Diatomaceous earth (diatomite)
This is a common ingredient in natural so-called wormers. It is a soft, chalky rock that gets its name from fossilized silica shell remains of diatoms, tiny marine phytoplankton. It is crushed into a fine powder.

Owing to its high content of crystalline silica, diatomite is mildly abrasive. Some grades of diatomite on the market may contain up to 60% of Crystalline silica. When inhaled Crystalline silica can cause the deadly silicosis.[145]

Diatomaceous earth is said to kill worms by slashing them with its blade-like surfaces. It is approved by the FDA for use in grain storage for preventing insect infestations.[146] However, there is not one single study that can attest to diatomaceous earth killing worms in horses. And if someone does believe that it does have a slasher-like effect on worms, then you would think they would feed a horse razor blades! Actually, the slasher-like effect is prevented by moisture, so as soon as the horse eats them, any sharp-edged effect is nullified. At any rate, there are two types of diatomaceous earth, food grade and industrial grade. Food grade only has a very mildly abrasive surface.

As I said, there is not one single scientific study that suggests diatomaceous earth will hurt horse worms in any way. Parasitologist J. Hoyt Snyder states, "'Alternative' dewormers have been touted in the organic press, but little evidence exists for efficacy even approaching that of the current generation of anthelmintics (at least for non-resistant parasites). Diatomaceous earth (DTE) is one of the more popular of these. Repeated efforts have been made to demonstrate some efficacy, but none have succeeded."[147]

Also, there are many studies that say diatomaceous earth is unsafe. Diatomaceous earth has been named as a serious respiratory hazard,[148] and chronic exposure to it causes fibrosis.[149]

I do not like to use chemical wormers, but I have no option as I also don't want my horses to die from worms. Let's say for argument's sake that herbal wormers do have some effect on certain horse worms.

Good. Yet the important thing is that only two chemicals of all the horse worming chemicals that are out there can be effective against the horse killer worms, encysted cyathostomes. Further, it does no good to experiment with giving herbal wormers to a group of horses and then doing Fecal Egg Counts, as egg counts cannot tell you anything about tapeworm or encysted cyathostome burden, and the only way to tell is, sad to say, on post mortem.

Copper as a dewormer

Myth

Horses with enough copper do not get worms.

Fact

No way! Wrong! There is not a drop of evidence to suggest this. I myself find it utterly reprehensible and highly irresponsible that anyone would suggest that optimal levels of copper in horses prevent horse worms, given the amount of painful awful deaths caused by worms. I myself personally knew a goat who was kept on high levels of copper by a natural therapist, a goat who died a slow death, and post mortem revealed an enormous worm burden. She was a show goat and had been looked after superbly (in other ways!), only her owner believed that copper would prevent worms. There is zero evidence for this – there is evidence that feeding copper needles may help with certain sheep worms, but zero for horse worms.

15. Fecal Egg Counts

Myth. Egg counts are a guide to the horse's worm infestation.
Facts. WRONG! WRONG! WRONG!
1) Egg counts do not show how badly a horse is infested with encysted small strongyles. This means the egg count could be clean of worms but the horse could be infested with these worms. [150] Egg counts cannot pick up encysted stages as they are in the lining of the intestine. Also, encysted small strongyle larvae are not mature enough to lay eggs. Yes, when they emerge from the intestine some of them will lay eggs, but by then it is too late for some horses! Plus they can stay encysted for years!

Eminent parasitologist Craig Reinemeyer stated, "It is a pervasive misconception that the objective of parasite control is to kill adult worms (i.e., the worms that lay the eggs detected by fecal examination). However, all strongyle parasites of horses exert their greatest pathogenicity in the larval stages that are by definition incapable of sexual reproduction."[151]

Repeat after me: Eggs of encysted small strongyles (cyathostomes) NEVER, yes, NEVER, NEVER, NEVER show up in Fecal Egg Counts!
Again, eggs of encysted small strongyles (cyathostomes) NEVER show up in Fecal Egg Counts! THEY DO NOT LAY EGGS!

2) Fecal Egg Counts cannot tell you the degree of parasite infestation in your horse. Not all worms lay eggs! Only the adult fertile, egg-laying, worms do, and get this, they don't even lay eggs consistently.

3) It takes a large number of egg-laying worms to return a positive Fecal Egg Count.

4) A Fecal Egg Count estimates the number of eggs in 1 gram of the horse's manure. It mainly detects eggs of adult roundworms, pinworms, large strongyles and small strongyles. It does not detect the presence of tapeworms (less than 3%),[152] bots, and the larval stages of any worms at all. By the time a Fecal Egg Count picks up the presence of *Strongylus vulgaris*, most of the damage has already been done. It is weeks or even months before the *Strongylus vulgaris* females return to the gut, mature, and then start laying eggs.[153] Likewise, Fecal Egg Counts are too late to be of any help with roundworms (*Parascaris equorum*), as tissue inflammation will already have occurred by the time these eggs show up.

5) As I said, egg counts tell you NOTHING about the degree of infestation of encysted small strongyles in a horse. Also, they cannot tell you much about the degree of tapeworm infestation in a horse. A horse can be full of tapeworms[154] and return a negative egg count.

This is important as it is overlooked by many articles even those written by some veterinary surgeons: A horse can be full of tapeworms and encysted small strongyles, even some other worms, and still return a negative egg count.

When Fecal Egg Counts are of vital importance

Fecal Egg Counts across your herd of horses or donkeys are necessary to show which individuals are more susceptible to worm burdens. A Fecal Egg Count will show which horses or donkeys are particularly susceptible to small strongyles. It is now recommended that it is only necessary to measure for strongyles once in a horse or donkey's lifetime, as the strongyle contaminative potential of the individual horse or donkey is genetically determined.[155]

You need to find out if your individual horse or donkey (not herd!) is genetically predisposed to small strongyles as this is what your worming regime should be based on.

16. Foals

Foals are susceptible to heavy burdens of ascarids and require a double dose of fenbendazole, and a double dose is also required to treat encysted early third stage, late third stage and fourth stage mucosal cyathostome larvae and fourth stage larvae of *Strongylus vulgaris* in all horses.[156]

You really need to be vigilant in worming foals. Last year I was speaking to a lady who had a foal just under four months old. This lady had been worming her horses with Equest (Quest), but had not done her foal, as she was waiting until he was older. As I had just bought in a large stock of Panacur 100, I offered to give her some, and instructed her to give it to the foal for 5 consecutive days. I went back the following day with my camera, and these are the results.

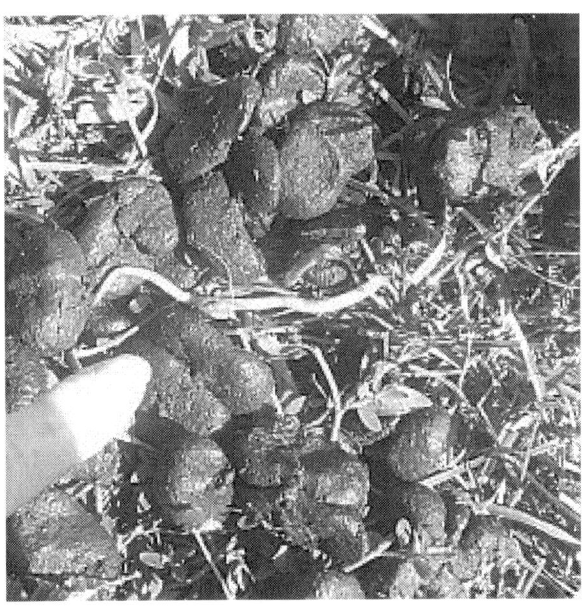

This is in fact typical of what will happen if you don't worm your foals. A fenbendazole wormer is a safe one to use for foals, who should be first treated at 4 weeks and then at 4-6 weekly intervals.[157] These photos show ascarids (*Parascaris equorum*). Different dewormers in different countries have different registered claims. The company that sells Quest (Equest) in the USA suggests deworming foals with their product initially at the age of 6 months of age, whereas in Australia, the suggestion is at 2 months.

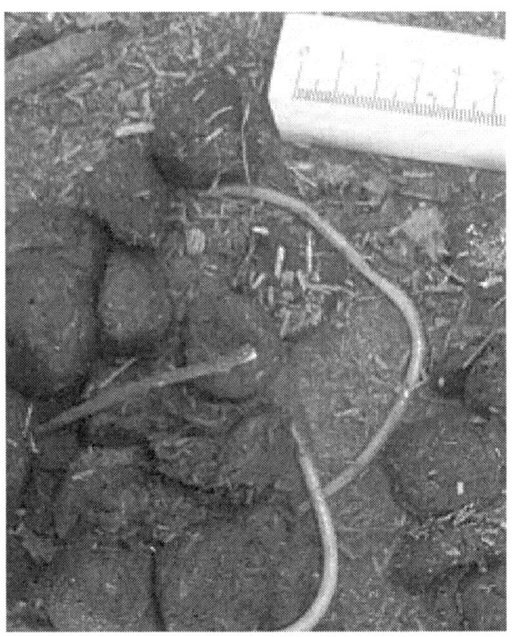

Now, for those people who really do believe that copper will prevent a horse getting worms, this foal and her mother were religiously fed 1 teaspoon of copper per day each in their feed, as their owner had read this recommendation in a book and followed it to the letter. Yes, horses do need copper (in the correct ratio –with zinc - to balance the iron in their feed), but it will not stop them getting worms!

17. Resistance and Rotation

Problems of resistance in small strongyles to benzimidazole have been widely documented worldwide[158] and have been reported as early as the 1960s.[159] Resistance to fenbendazole, mebendazole, febantel, and oxibendazole has been reported,[160] as has resistance to pyrantel,[161] and more recently to ivermectin[162] and moxidectin.[163] Interestingly, one instance of moxidectin resistance was reported in donkeys.[164] Roundworms have recently found to demonstrate resistance to ivermectin.[165]

The cause has been associated with irregular worming intervals or with non rotation of different classes of dewormer for long periods of time.[166] Rotation, as well as overuse of dewormers, also contributes to resistance.[167]

Rotation used to be, and unfortunately often still is, widely advocated as the cure-all for worm resistance. Slow and fast rotation schemes have been put forward, as have other rotational schemes, but there have been very few studies on such schemes.

Changing wormer chemical classes frequently contributes to resistance, as does underdosing. In the 1980s, Professor Reuben Rose (former Chair at the University of Sydney Department of Veterinary Science and Head of their Equine Exercise Physiology Unit) was to the forefront of horse worm research for some years, and said rotation of drug groups must not be done more than once a year as it causes resistance.[168] Pathobiologist and worm researcher Andrew S. Peregrine states, "Because this resistance appears to have arisen in association with excessive and inappropriate use of dewormers, there is increasingly a need for veterinarians to look critically at the deworming programs used by clients so that problems with anthelmintic resistance do not worsen."[169]

Recent research, reported in 2008, stated, "For several decades, equine anthelmintic programs have focused on rotational deworming strategies in which horses are dewormed with different anthelmintic classes separated by predictable intervals. This approach is no longer sustainable because rotation does not slow, and in fact, it actually selects for resistance to all drugs in the rotation."[170] The research stated that rotational schemes may mask anthelmintic resistance by the regular substitution of effective products in the deworming schedule. These days, slow rotation, in which a single dewormer is used for an entire year, is a particular concern due to resistance among small strongyles. Worms that are sensitive to a particular anthelmintic are killed, while the resistant parasites live on happily for a lengthy period of time and come to dominate the population.[171]

The prevalence of pyrantel resistance[172] in North America is significantly higher than other parts of the world.[173] Daily dosing of low-dose pyrantel is not licensed in most other parts of the world, and the evidence suggests that the daily feeding has caused resistance.[174]

A study reported in 2006 on the effects of fenbendazole on parasite resistance[175] concluded that neither dosage every 28 days nor larger doses of fenbendazole reduced fenbendazole resistance. The study demonstrated that fenbendazole resistance in a group of horses can be reduced or broken by rotation of anthelmintic classes. The study also concluded that further research is needed to evaluate all aspects of rotation in the horse, and recommended that comparisons of fast and slow rotation should be carried out in order to determine how we can slow the problem of parasite resistance and how each class of anthelmintic can be used to the best effect.[176]

However, Reinemeyer points out that rotation is no longer an option, because only one chemical class (macrocyclic lactones, for example moxidectin and ivermectin) are consistently effective against cyathostomes.[177] He also states, "Future approaches to equine parasite control … and using anthelmintic treatments much less frequently and only in selected members of a herd."[178]

To put it in a nutshell, in the old days, the idea was to rotate. Now, the research indicates to worm horses or donkeys as individuals and not as a herd, and to take into account the genetic predisposition to strongyles of the individual, and to worm at certain times of year with certain products depending on your geographical location. Go to chapter 19, "When to worm and what with."

18. Prevention

Prevention of worm infestation is more important than ever with the increasing resistance to anthelmintics. The first thing to do is to remove manure. Studies have shown how effective removal of manure is in keeping worm burdens to a minimum.[179] It has the added benefit of increasing the grazing area. If can afford a pasture vacuum, you're in luck! However, if you feel like some of us with what seems to be a never ending supply of manure, just do the best you can – some removal is actually better than none! If your horses are not on total grazing, start by removing the manure around the feed areas.

Now if you have stables and don't clean them out as often as you should, you're also in luck as ammonia from filthy dirty wet stables (sound familiar?) will kill nematode larvae.[180] Stall environments, even clean ones, are not good for worms, and strongyles are almost entirely picked up from pasture.[181]

Horses become infected with cyathostomes by eating infective larvae in pasture. It's therefore a good idea not to have manure lying around paddocks, and it's certainly not a good idea to throw hay on top of it.

Dung beetles are a good friend to the horse owner, so try not to kill the little critters. Overgrazing means the manure is quickly trodden down, and this is not good for dung beetles. Studies have shown moxidectin (another good reason to use Equest/Quest!) does not harm dung beetles.[182] Dung beetles increase soil fertility, soil aeration, and water infiltration into the soil. Dung beetles bury nutrients into the soil.[183] They get rid of manure, which is good in itself but also helps against horse worms. No wonder the ancient Egyptians were so fond of them!

Worm eggs and larvae can survive very cold weather, but larvae are killed by hot, dry conditions. Of course, there is nothing you can do about the weather, but this is good to know. Be more vigilant if you are from a cold climate.

Harrowing pasture

Harrowing is often suggested as a preventative measure for worm control but in fact it actually increases worms. Horses with plenty of room on which to graze will divide their grazing into two distinct areas, 1) roughs and 2) lawns. They do nearly all their droppings in the rough area, an area with overgrown grass and weeds, an area which horses will not graze down. The lawns are the areas which horses do graze, and on which they rarely do droppings. Clearly then, most of the worm eggs are in the roughs.[184] This is a natural system for horses to keep down their worm burdens.

Harrowing, mowing or dragging comprises this system. Harrowing, mowing or dragging transfers the high levels of worm eggs from the roughs to the lawns.

Harrowing, mowing or dragging increases worm levels by transferring the high levels of worm eggs from the 'roughs' to the 'lawns.'

If done at all, harrowing or mowing should be carried out at the hottest time of year, and the horses should then be kept off the area for several weeks. However, in cooler regions, harrowing at the end of the grazing season has been shown to reduce the survival of infective stages of worms over winter.[185]

19. When to worm and what with?

Ambient temperature has a foremost impact on the load of infective worm larvae in the environment.[186] L3 small strongyle (cyathostome) larvae have a cuticle that prevents them ingesting nutrients. When ambient temperatures exceed 85°F (29.5° C), the heightened L3 activity along with the absence of nutrient ingestion leads to the death of larvae which of course means a seasonal decrease in infective L3 on the pasture. It also would make sense that this would reduce the need for deworming. This is particularly important when taking into account the little critters known as refugia.

Refugia

What are refugia? Refugia are the key to preventing resistance to dewormers. Parasitologists Swiderski and French state, "The major unifying goal in preventing anthelmintic resistance is to increase the frequency of anthelmintic-susceptible parasites in the environment."[187] Refugia are worms which are lacking in genetic resistance to dewormers, basically as they have not been exposed to them when the horse was wormed – either by being encysted, or on the ground waiting for a horse to eat them. The more of these refugia in the horse population, the better. (Not that more worms are good of course, but if horses do have worms, it is better that they have worms with no genetic resistance to dewormers!) The less frequently the horse is wormed, the more refugia are present.

Seasonal

So when the ambient temperatures exceed 85°F (29.5° C), less refugia are on pasture and deworming at this time will seriously pressure the refugia, not a good thing.[188] Seasonal conditions that favor peak fecal egg production also favor pasture contamination and larger refugia populations. More frequent deworming is recommended at this time.

In warm temperate and subtropical and tropical climates, numbers of infective strongyle L3 on pasture drop dramatically during the summer, and this means that there is a time of grazing that is relatively free of exposure to small strongyles.[189] On the other hand, peak fecal egg production occurs from fall (autumn) through to spring.[190]

Bear in mind that infective L3 larvae are present on pastures in the warm temperate, subtropical, and tropical regions throughout the winter months. In cool and cool temperate regions, infective L3 are at their lowest during the winter but live through the winter to be present on pastures during spring, summer, and fall (autumn).[191] Fall (autumn) is an ideal time to deworm with a combination of macrocyclic lactone and praziquantel for encysted cyathostomes, tapeworms and bots.

Eggs are not likely to hatch and larvae are unlikely to develop in cold winter temperatures below 45°F (7°C). However, as noted above, already developed L3 will carry on in these temperatures for the season and will be a source of infection in spring grazing.[192]

Egg Reappearance Period (ERP)

Egg Reappearance Period is the length of time a horse's droppings will remain free of strongyle eggs after being dewormed. This is of great help in determining when to worm for strongyles. If you use a wormer at times which coincide with the egg reappearance period, you are likely to suppress egg contamination and thus suppress environmental contamination.[193]

Here are the reported ERPs for various anthelmintics.

Benzimidazole	2 weeks[194] to 4 weeks[195]
Fenbendazole	4 weeks[196]
Oxibendazole	4 weeks[197]
Pyrantel pamoate	4-6 weeks[198]
Ivermectin	6 weeks[199] to 8 weeks[200]
Moxidectin	12 weeks[201]

Note that in horses under the age of three, egg reappearance periods can be 25 – 40% shorter.[202]

Individual susceptibility
As noted previously, some horses are more susceptible to worm burdens than others. Parasitologists Swiderski and French state, "Therefore, the timehonored principle of simultaneous anthelmintic treatment of all herd mates is being rewritten to characterize the strongyle susceptibility of all herd mates."[203] They suggest that only those horses with a moderate to high susceptibility to strongyle infestation should be wormed when they have high Fecal Egg Counts.

They also note that if a herd is tested for Fecal Egg Counts, these individuals will show a higher count.[204] Remember that in the chapter on Fecal Egg Counts, we saw that it is only necessary to measure for strongyles once in a horse or donkey's lifetime, as strongyle susceptibility of the individual horse or donkey is genetically determined.[205] Some horses have an ability to control strongyle infections in the absence of chemical dewormers, and these horses should not be wormed as frequently as other members of the herd.[206]

When to worm and what with? The bottom line
Rotation is no longer the answer. The current research says that we are to consider our own climate, and the individual horse or donkey, and not worm the whole herd at the same time like we all used to do.

Rotation is no longer the answer. The current research says that we are to consider the individual horse or donkey and not worm the whole herd at the same time like we all used to do.

Foals should be treated for roundworms at 2 months of age, and then do a Fecal Egg Count 2 months later. If it says roundworms are present then, worm again, if not, do not worm.

Bots can be treated in autumn or early winter, and this is also (in many climates) a good time to treat for encysted cyathostomes. So, either moxidectin, or fenbendazole plus something that will treat bots.

Reinemeyer states that it is unnecessary to worm horses in the 6 month period in one's own geographical location at the time unfavorable for strongyle transmission, as the climate rather than a chemical takes care of the worms.[207]

20. When to worm according to your climate

It must be stressed that these charts[208] are a GUIDE only. They do not take into account horses with an encysted cyathostome problem – deal with this problem before being guided by the following charts.

The geographic regions are approximate only – sub-regions may differ greatly.

Just remember that these are the unfavorable conditions for cyathostomes to lay eggs and thus these are the times to avoid worming:
1) Cold winter areas:
Late fall (autumn) or early winter
OR
2) Mild winter areas with hot summers:
Summer.

Chart 1: Northern hemisphere (cold winters)
Example: Eastern North America at latitudes between 40 and 60° north.
Northern Europe including the middle latitudes of European Russia; north-eastern China, Russian Dongbei, Korea, Japan;
Much of the USA
Much of Canada including the eastern provinces.
UK
Much of Western Europe
Much of northwest Europe
Steppes of Russia and the Ukraine,
Prairies of Canada and the USA

Chart 2: Northern hemisphere (mild winters and hot summers)
Example: Florida, USA.
southeastern China

Chart 3: Southern hemisphere (cold winters)
Example: Australia: Tasmania, Canberra, New England (NSW) region, the high country of Victoria, the alpine region of NSW

Chart 4: Southern hemisphere (mild winters and hot summers)
Example: Australia: Melbourne, Adelaide (Australia) most of southern, and South East coastal Zones.
New Zealand, southern South America and South Africa.

Chart 1: Northern hemisphere

Strongyle Contaminative Potential of individual horse	March-April	+ 2 months (May or June)	+ 3 months (June or July)	+4 months (July or August)	+6 months (September or October)
Low	Ivermectin & Praziquantel ***Or*** Moxidectin & Praziquantel (**or** Fenbendazole plus Praziquantel product)				Moxidectin & Praziquantel (**or** Fenbendazole plus Praziquantel product) ***Or*** Ivermectin & Praziquantel
Moderate	Ivermectin & Praziquantel ………….. ***Or*** Moxidectin & Praziquantel (**or** Fenbendazole plus Praziquantel product)	BZ or Pyrantel …………..	Do not worm …………… BZ or Pyrantel		Moxidectin & Praziquantel (**or** Fenbendazole plus Praziquantel product) ***Or*** Ivermectin & Praziquantel
High	Ivermectin & Praziquantel …………….. ***Or*** Moxidectin & Praziquantel (**or** Fenbendazole plus Praziquantel product)	BZ or Pyrantel ……………	Ivermectin or Moxidectin ……………. BZ or Pyrantel	Do not worm ……….. Ivermectin	Moxidectin & Praziquantel (**or** Fenbendazole plus Praziquantel product) ***Or*** Ivermectin & Praziquantel

BZ product = Oxibendazole, Fenbendazole, Mebendazole, or Oxfendazole

Chart 2: Northern hemisphere

Strongyle Contaminative Potential of individual horse	September-October	+ 2 months (November or December)	+ 3 months (December or January)	+4 months (January or February)	+6 months (March or April)
Low	Ivermectin & Praziquantel ***Or*** Moxidectin & Praziquantel (**or** Fenbendazole plus Praziquantel product)				Moxidectin & Praziquantel (**or** Fenbendazole plus Praziquantel product) ***Or*** Ivermectin & Praziquantel
Moderate	Ivermectin & Praziquantel .... ***Or*** Moxidectin & Praziquantel (**or** Fenbendazole plus Praziquantel product)	BZ or Pyrantel	Do not worm .... BZ or Pyrantel		Moxidectin & Praziquantel .... (**or** Fenbendazole plus Praziquantel product) ***Or*** Ivermectin & Praziquantel
High	Ivermectin & Praziquantel .... ***Or*** Moxidectin & Praziquantel (**or** Fenbendazole plus Praziquantel product)	BZ or Pyrantel .... Do not worm	Ivermectin or Moxidectin .... BZ or Pyrantel		Moxidectin & Praziquantel .... (**or** Fenbendazole plus Praziquantel product) ***Or*** Ivermectin & Praziquantel

Chart 3: Southern hemisphere

Strongyle Contaminative Potential of individual horse	September-October	+ 2 months (November or December)	+ 3 months (December or January)	+4 months (January or February)	+6 months (March or April)
Low	Ivermectin & Praziquantel ***Or*** Moxidectin & Praziquantel (**or** Fenbendazole plus Praziquantel product)				Moxidectin & Praziquantel (**or** Fenbendazole plus Praziquantel product) ***Or*** Ivermectin & Praziquantel
Moderate	Ivermectin & Praziquantel …………… ***Or*** Moxidectin & Praziquantel (**or** Fenbendazole plus Praziquantel product)	BZ or Pyrantel ……………	Do not worm …………… BZ or Pyrantel		Moxidectin & Praziquantel ………… (**or** Fenbendazole plus Praziquantel product) ***Or*** Ivermectin & Praziquantel
High	Ivermectin & Praziquantel …………… ***Or*** Moxidectin & Praziquantel (**or** Fenbendazole plus Praziquantel product)	BZ or Pyrantel …………… Do not worm	Ivermectin or Moxidectin ………… BZ or Pyrantel		Moxidectin & Praziquantel ………… (**or** Fenbendazole plus Praziquantel product) ***Or*** Ivermectin & Praziquantel

Chart 4 : Southern hemisphere

Strongyle Contaminative Potential of individual horse	March-April	+ 2 months (May or June)	+ 3 months (June or July)	+4 months (July or August)	+6 months (September or October)
Low	Ivermectin & Praziquantel ***Or*** Moxidectin & Praziquantel (**or** Fenbendazole plus Praziquantel product)				Moxidectin & Praziquantel (**or** Fenbendazole plus Praziquantel product) ***Or*** Ivermectin & Praziquantel
Moderate	Ivermectin & Praziquantel ………….. ***Or*** Moxidectin & Praziquantel (**or** Fenbendazole plus Praziquantel product)	BZ or Pyrantel …………..	Do not worm …………… BZ or Pyrantel		Moxidectin & Praziquantel (**or** Fenbendazole plus Praziquantel product) ***Or*** Ivermectin & Praziquantel
High	Ivermectin & Praziquantel …………….. ***Or*** Moxidectin & Praziquantel (**or** Fenbendazole plus Praziquantel product)	BZ or Pyrantel ……………	Ivermectin or Moxidectin ……………. BZ or Pyrantel	Do not worm ……….. Ivermectin	Moxidectin & Praziquantel (**or** Fenbendazole plus Praziquantel product) ***Or*** Ivermectin & Praziquantel

Appendix: Worming Products.[209]

Product	Active Ingredients	Small strongyles	Large strongyles	Ascarids	Intestinal Threadworms	Hairworms	Stomach Worms	Pinworms	Lungworms	Tapeworms	Bots	Encysted Cyathostomes
Equest Plus Tape / Quest Plus / Equest Pramox	moxidectin and praziquantel	■	■	■	■	■	■	■	■	■	■	■
Equest / Quest / Equest Oral Gel	moxidectin	■	■	■	■	■	■	■	■		■	■
Equitape	Praziquantel									■		
Equimax Paste USA, UK, Europe	Ivermectin and Praziquantel	■	■	■	■	■	■	■	■	■	■	
Equimax Paste Australia	Abamectin and Praziquantel	■	■	■	■	■	■	■	■	■	■	
Eraquell	Ivermectin	■	■	■	■	■	■	■	■		■	

Product	Active Ingredients	Small strongyles	Large strongyles	Ascarids	Intestinal Threadworms	Hairworms	Stomach Worms	Pinworms	Lungworms	Tapeworms	Bots	Encysted Cyathostomes
Eqvalan	Ivermectin											
Eqvalan Duo / Eqvalan Gold	Ivermectin and Praziquantel											
Strongid-P /Strongid (Granules liquid & Paste)	Pyrantel Embonate											
Panacur / Pancur Paste	Fenbendazole											
Exodus	Pyrantel Pamoate									* *		
Safeguard	Fenbendazole											
Equimec	Ivermectin											

** Effective against some tapeworms at double dose.

Product	Active Ingredients	Small strongyles	Large strongyles	Ascarids	Intestinal Threadworms	Hairworms	Stomach Worms	Pinworms	Lungworms	Tapeworms	Bots	Encysted Cyathostomes
Pyratape P	Pyrantel Embonate											
Noromet cin	Ivermectin											
Telmin (Granules & Paste)	Mebendazole								X			
Vectin	Ivermectin											
Bimectin	Ivermectin											
Equell	Ivermectin											
Valumec	Abamectin											

X Donkeys with lungworms will need higher dose over 5 days.

Product	Active Ingredients	Small strongyles	Large strongyles	Ascarids	Intestinal Threadworms	Hairworms	Stomach Worms	Pinworms	Lungworms	Tapeworms	Bots	Encysted Cyathostomes
Embotape	Pyrantel Embonate									**X**		
Zimecterin	Ivermectin											
Zimecterin Gold	Ivermectin and Praziquantel											
Anthelcide	Oxibendazole											
Farnam Continuex Daily Dewormer	Pyrantel tartrate											
CW Continuous Wormer	Pyrantel tartrate											
Systamex	Oxfendazole											

X At double dose

Product	Active Ingredients	Small strongyles	Large strongyles	Ascarids	Intestinal Threadworms	Hairworms	Stomach Worms	Pinworms	Lungworms	Tapeworms	Bots	Encysted Cyathostomes
Strongyle Care	Pyrantel Pamoate	■	■	■				■				
Ivercare	Ivermectin	■	■	■	■	■	■	■	■		■	
Safe-Guard Equi-Bits	Fenbendazole	■	■	■	■			■				■
Safe-Guard Equine Paste	Fenbendazole	■	■	■	■			■				■
Strongid C	Pyrantel tartrate	■	■	■				■				
Rotectin P	Pyrantel tartrate	■	■	■				■				
Valumec Ivermectin Liquid	Ivermectin	■	■	■	■	■	■	■	■		■	

Product	Active Ingredients	Small strongyles	Large strongyles	Ascarids	Intestinal Threadworms	Hairworms	Stomach Worms	Pinworms	Lungworms	Tapeworms	Bots	Encysted Cyathostomes
TapcCare Plus	Pyrantel Pamoate											
Equi-Aid CW	Pyrantel Tartrate											
Expel - Yellow Tube	Abamectin and Morantel Tartrate											
Ammo	Abamectin and Morantel Tartrate											
Farnam MecWorma & Tape	Abamectin and Morantel Tartrate											
Promectin Plus	Abamectin and Praziquantel											
Eraquell Pellets	Ivermectin											

Product	Active Ingredients	Small strongyles	Large strongyles	Ascarids	Intestinal Threadworms	Hairworms	Stomach Worms	Pinworms	Lungworms	Tapeworms	Bots	Encysted Cyathostomes
Equimax Elevation	Pyrantel Embonate, Praziquantel & Ivermectin.											
Valumax - Red Tube	Abamectin and Praziquantel											
Equimax LV (Australia)	Abamectin and Praziquantel											
Farnam MecWorma & Bot	Abamectin											
Razor	Ivermectin and Praziquantel											
Imax Gold	Ivermectin and Praziquantel											
Equimec Plus Tape	Ivermectin and Praziquantel											

Product	Active Ingredients	Small strongyles	Large strongyles	Ascarids	Intestinal Threadworms	Hairworms	Stomach Worms	Pinworms	Lungworms	Tapeworms	Bots	Encysted Cyathostomes
Evolve	Ivermectin and Praziquantel	■	■	■	■	■	■	■	■	■	■	
Genesis	Ivermectin and Praziquantel	■	■	■	■	■	■	■	■	■	■	
Equimec Plus Tape	Ivermectin and Praziquantel	■	■	■	■	■	■	■	■	■	■	
Outback Vet Allwormer Paste	Ivermectin and Praziquantel	■	■	■	■	■	■	■	■	■	■	
Equiban (Granules & paste)	Morantel tartrate	■	■	■				■		■		
Strategy T	Oxfendazole and Pyrantel Embonate	■	■	■				■		■		
Oximinth Paste	Oxibendazole	■	■	■				■				

Product	Active Ingredients	Small strongyles	Large strongyles	Ascarids	Intestinal Threadworms	Hairworms	Stomach Worms	Pinworms	Lungworms	Tapeworms	Bots	Encysted Cyathostomes
Equinox-Orange Tube	Oxfendazole	■	■	■		■	■	■				
Farnam Worma Paste	Oxfendazole and Piperazine	■	■	■		■	■	■				
Farnam Worms Drench	Oxfendazole	■	■	■		■	■	■				
Oximinth Plus Paste	Oxibendazole and dichlorvos	■	■	■				■			■	
Valumec – Green Tube	Abamectin	■	■	■	■	■	■	■	■		■	
Farnam ComboCare	Moxidectin and praziquantel	■	■	■	■	■	■	■	■	■	■	■

Endnotes

1 Drudge, JH, Lyons, ET. "Control of internal parasites of the horse." *J Am Vet Med Assoc (Journal of the American Veterinary Medical Association*)1966;148:378-383.

2 In Australia however, this is the (single) recommended dose.

3 Samson-Himmelstjerna von G, Fritzen B, Demeler J, Schurmann S, Rohn K, Schnieder T, Epe C, "Cases of reduced cyathostomin egg reappearance period and failure of Parascaris equorum egg count reduction following ivermectin treatment as well as survey on pyrantel efficacy on German horse farms." *Vet. Parasitol.* (*Veterinary Parasitology*) 2007; 144: 74-80; Doorn van DCK, Lems S, Weteling A, Ploeger HW, Eysker M, "Resistance of Parascaris equorum against ivermectin due to frequent anthelmintic treatment of foals in the Netherlands," *20th International Conference of the WAAVP*, Gent, 2007; Hearn F.P.D, Peregrine A.S., "Identification of foals infected with Parascaris equorum apparently resistant to ivermectin." *JAVMA* (*Journal of the American Veterinary Medical Association)* 2003; 223: 482-85; Stoneham S, Coles GC, "Ivermectin resistance in Parascaris equorum," *Vet.Rec.* (*The Veterinary Record*) 2006; 158:572; Boersema JH, Borgsteede FHM, Eysker M, Elema TE, Gaasenbeek CPH and Burg van der WPJ, "The prevalence of anthelmintic resistance of horse strongyles in the Netherlands," *Vet. Quart.* (*Veterinary Quarterly*) 1991; 13: 209-17; Boersema JH, Eysker M, Maas J and Aar van der WM, "Comparison of the reappearance of strongyle eggs in foals, yearlings, and adult horses after treatment with ivermectin or pyrantel," *Vet. Quart.* 1996 18: 7-9; Deborah C.K. van Doorn and Harm W. Ploeger, "Worming horses the rational way," *European Veterinary Conference* Voorjaarsdagen Amsterdam, Netherlands 2008; Kaplan RM, "Anthelmintic resistance in nematodes of horses," *Vet Res* (*Veterinary Research*) 2002; 33:491–507; Coles GC, Jackson F, Pomroy WE, *et al.* "The

detection of anthelmintic resistance in nematodes of veterinary importance. *Vet Parasitol* 2006;136:167–185.

[4] Noritaka Hirazawa, Taro Ohtaka and Kazuhiko Hata, "Challenge trials on the anthelmintic effect of drugs and natural agents against the monogenean Heterobothrium okamotoi in the tiger puffer Takifugu rubripes." *Aquaculture*, Volume 188, Issues 1-2, 1 August 2000, 1-13.

[5] Barbara J Fougère; Susan G Wynn, *Veterinary Herbal Medicine*, St. Louis : Mosby, an affiliate of Elsevier, 2007. p. 430.

[6] Lankas, G.R and Gordon L.R.. Toxicology in W.C. Campbell (ed.). 1989; "Ivermectin and Abamectin." Springer-Verlag, NY; Hayes, W.J. and E.R. Laws (eds.). 1990. *Handbook of Pesticide Toxicology, Classes of Pesticides*, Vol. 3. Academic Press, Inc., NY.

[7] Hayes, W.J. and E.R. Laws (eds.). 1990. *Handbook of Pesticide Toxicology, Classes of Pesticides*, Vol. 3. Academic Press, Inc., NY.

[8] Purdy S.R. "Herd Health for Miniature Donkeys," In: *Veterinary Care of Donkeys*, Matthews N.S. and Taylor T.S. (Eds.). International Veterinary Information Service, Ithaca NY (www.ivis.org), Last updated: 1-Apr-2005; A2921.0405

[9] Anne Courroucé-Malblanc, G. Fortier, M. Moulin, J. J.P. Valette, L. Petit, S. Dumontier, P.H. Pitel, "Reference Values on Hematologic and Biochemical Parameters in French Donkeys," *Proceedings of the 10th International Congress of World Equine Veterinary Association.* 2008 - Moscow, Russia.

[10] Duncan, J.L., Pirie, H.M., "The life cycle of Strongylus vulgaris in the horse," *Res Vet Sci.* (*Research in Veterinary Science*) 1972 Jul;13(4):374-9.

[11] Murray, M. J. "Treatment of Equine Gastrointestinal Parasites," In: *8ème Congrès de médecine et chirurgie équine - 8. Kongress für Pferdemedezin und -chirurgie - 8th Congress on Equine Medicine and Surgery*, 2003 - Geneva, Switzerland, Chuit P., Kuffer A. and Montavon S. (Eds.) International Veterinary Information Service, Ithaca NY (www.ivis.org), 2003; P0727.1203.

[12] C. Monahan, "Anthelmintic Control Strategies for Horses,"

in *Companion and Exotic Animal Parasitology*, Bowman D.D. (Ed.), International Veterinary Information Service, Ithaca NY 2000; A0309.0500.

13 "Exsheath."

14 McCraw B. M. and Slocombe J. O. D. "Early Development of and Pathology Associated with Strongylus edentatus," *Can J Comp Med.* (*Canadian Journal of Comparative Medicine and Veterinary Science*) 1974 April; 38(2): 124–138.

15 McCraw B M and Slocombe J O, "Strongylus equinus: development and pathological effects in the equine host," *Can J Comp Med.* 1985 October; 49(4): 372–383; Murray, M.J. *Ibid.*

16 K. Lindgrena, Ö. Ljungvallb, O. Nilssonc, B.-L. Ljungströmd, C. Lindahla and J. Höglund, "Parascaris equorum in foals and in their environment on a Swedish stud farm, with notes on treatment failure of ivermectin," *Veterinary Parasitology*, Volume 151, Issues 2-4, 14 February 2008, 337-343.

17 Murray, M.J. *Ibid.*

18 *Loc. cit.*

19 *Loc. cit.*

20 P.A. Payne and G.R. Carter, "Parasitic Diseases: Arthropods," *A Concise Guide to the Microbial and Parasitic Diseases of Horses*, Carter G.R., Payne P.A. and Davis E. (Eds.). International Veterinary Information Service, Ithaca NY (www.ivis.org), Last updated: 27-Mar-2008.

21 Murray, M.J. *Ibid.*

22 Ogbourne CP. "Observations on the free-living stages of strongylid nematodes of the horse." *Parasitology* 1972;64: 461–477; Rupasinghe D, Ogbourne CP. Laboratory studies on the effect of temperature on the development of the free-living stages of some strongylid nematodes of the horse. *Z Parasitenk* (*ZEITSCHRIFT FUR PFLANZENERNAHRUNG UND BODENKUNDE*) 1978; 55:249–253.

23 C.R. Reinemeyer, "Controlling Strongyle Parasites of Horses: A Mandate for Change," Proceedings of the 55th Annual Convention of the American Association of Equine Practitioners, 2009.

24 Murray, M.J. *Ibid.*

[25] Smith HJ. "Strongyle infections in ponies. I. Response to intermittent thiabendazole treatment." *Can J Comp Med* 1976;40:327–333.

[26] http://www.fda.gov/cvm/FOI/141-087s112305.pdf

[27] P. Dorchies, "Anthelmintic Resistance and Control of Roundworms," *Proceedings of the 9th International Congress of World Equine Veterinary Association* 2006, Morocco.

[28] Joseph A. DiPietro, DVM, MS; Thomas Klei, PhD; and Craig Reinemeyer, DVM, PhD, "Efficacy of Fenbendazole Against Encysted Small Strongyle Larvae," *Proceedings of the Annual Convention of the AAEP*, 1997, 343-344. However, resistance has now been demonstrated, cf. Murray, M.J. *Ibid.*

[29] NADA 120-648 Panacur and Safe-Guard - supplemental approval (May 28, 1985)

[30] Andrew S. Peregrine, "Deworming programs for horses: are we doing more harm than good?" *As Presented in the Rounds of Department of Large Animal Clinical Sciences Western College of Veterinary Medicine*, June/July 2005, Vol. 5, Issue 6; Giles CJ, Urquhart KA, Longstaffe JA, "Larval cyathostomosiasis (immature trichostronema-induced enteropathy): a report of 15 clinical cases." *Equine Veterinary Journal* 1985;17:196–201; Love S, Murphy D, Mellor D., "Pathogenicity of cyathostome infection," *Vet Parasitol* (1999) 85:113-121; Slocombe, JOD, De Gannes, R., "Effectiveness of moxidectin for benzimidazole and pyrantel resistant cyathostomes in horses," *Proceedings, 43rd Annual Meeting of the American Association of Veterinary Parasitologists* 1998:53; Peregrine A, McEwen B, Lusis P, *et al.*, "Larval cyathostomiasis in horses: a new disease in Ontario?" *Animal Health Laboratory Newsletter*, University of Guelph 2002;6:22.

[31] Tarigo-Martinie, JL, Wyatt, AR, Kaplan, RM., "Prevalence, clinical implications of anthelmintic resistance in cyathostomes of horses," *J Am Vet Med Assoc (Journal of the American Veterinary Medical Association*) 2001; 218, 1957-1960.

[32] Baudena, MA, Chapman, MR, Horohov, DW, *et al.* "Protective responses against cyathostome infections." *Proceedings of the 19th International WAAVP Conf*, 2003.

[33] Murray, M.J. *Ibid.*

[34] C.R. Reinemeyer, "Controlling Strongyle Parasites of Horses: A Mandate for Change," *Proceedings of the 55th Annual Convention of the American Association of Equine Practitioners*, 2009.

[35] Giles CJ, Urquhart KA, Longstaffe JA., "Larval cyathostomosiasis (immature trichostronema-induced enteropathy): a report of 15 clinical cases," *Equine Veterinary Journal* 1985;17:196–201.

[36] *Loc. cit.* http://72.14.235.132/search?q=cache:BhODK4SLdIUJ:www.wyethah.ca/pdfs/quest_parasite.pps+encysted+cyathostomes+do+not+lay+eggs&cd=1&hl=en&ct=clnk.

[37] Hodgkinson JE "Cyathostomosis: Epidemiology and control," *Proceedings of the 47th British Equine Veterinary Association Congress* 2008; Joseph A. DiPietro, DVM, MS; Thomas Klei, PhD; and Craig Reinemeyer, DVM, PhD, "Efficacy of Fenbendazole Against Encysted Small Strongyle Larvae," *Proceedings of the Annual Convention of the AAEP* (1997) Vol. 43, 343-343, see at http://www.ivis.org/proceedings/aaep/1997/Dipietro.pdf

[38] Hodgkinson JE, *Ibid.*

[39] Joseph A. DiPietro, DVM, MS; Thomas Klei, PhD; and Craig Reinemeyer, DVM, PhD, "Efficacy of Fenbendazole Against Encysted Small Strongyle Larvae," *Proceedings of the Annual Convention of the AAEP* (1997) Vol. 43, 343-343, see at http://www.ivis.org/proceedings/aaep/1997/Dipietro.pdf

[40] ivis.org/proceedings/aaep/1997/Dipietro.pdf

[40] Hodgkinson JE, *Ibid.*

[41] Reid SWJ, Mair TS, Hillyer MH, Love S. "Epidemiological risk factors associated with a diagnosis of clinical cyathostomiasis in the horse." *Equine Vet J* (*Equine Veterinary Journal*) 1995; 27: 127-130; Giles CJ, Urquhart KA, Longstaffe JA. "Larval cyathostomiasis (immature trichonema-induced enteropathy): A report of 15 clinical cases." *Equine Vet J* 1985; 17: 196-201; Paul JW. "Equine larval cyathostomosis." *Comp Cont Edu Pract Vet* (*Compendium on Continuing Education for the Practicing Veterinarian*) 1998; 20: 509-513.

42 C. Monahan, "Anthelmintic Control Strategies for Horses," in *Companion and Exotic Animal Parasitology*, Bowman D.D. (Ed.), International Veterinary Information Service, Ithaca NY 2000; A0309.0500.

43 *Loc. cit.*

44 Love S, Murphy D, Mellor D., "Pathogenicity of cyathostomes infection," *Vet Parasitol* (1999) 85:113-121.

45 Gomez HH, Georgi JR. "Equine helminth infections: control by selective chemotherapy." *Equine Vet J* 1991;23:198–200; See also Nielsen MK, Haaning N, Olsen SN. "Strongyle egg shedding consistency in horses on farms using selective therapy in Denmark." *Vet Parasitol* 2006;135:333–335; Dopfer D, Kerssens CM, Meijer YG, *et al*. "Shedding consistency of strongyle-type eggs in Dutch boarding horses." *Vet Parasitol* 2004;124:249–258.

46 Dr Christine King BVSc, MACVSc, MVetClinStud, *Natural Dewormers*, at http://www.animavet.com/NaturalDewormers.pdf. See also Swiderski, C.E. and French, D.D., "Paradigms for Parasite Control in Adult Horse Populations: A Review." *54th Annual Convention of the American Association of Equine Practitioners - AAEP*, 2008 - San Diego, CA, USA; Nielsen MK, Haaning N, Olsen SN. Strongyle egg shedding consistency in horses on farms using selective therapy in Denmark. *Vet Parasitol* 2006;135:333–335; Uhlinger CA. "Uses of Fecal Egg Count data in equine practice." *Comp Cont Educ Pract Vet* 1993;15:742–749.

47 Joseph A. DiPietro, DVM, MS; Thomas Klei, PhD; and Craig Reinemeyer, DVM, PhD, "Efficacy of Fenbendazole Against Encysted Small Strongyle Larvae," *Proceedings of the Annual Convention of the AAEP* (1997) Vol. 43, 343-343, see at http://www.ivis.org/proceedings/aaep/1997/Dipietro.pdf

48 Ray M. Kaplan, DVM, PhD, Thomas R. Klei, PhD Eugene T. Lyons, PhD, Guy Lester, DVM, PhD, Charles H. Courtney, DVM, PhD Dennis D. French, DVM, Sharon C. Tolliver, MS. N. Vidyashankar, PhD, Ying Zhao, MS, "Prevalence of anthelmintic resistant cyathostomes on horse farms," *Journal of the American Veterinary Medical Association*, September 15, 2004, Vol. 225, No. 6, 903-910.

49 NADA 120-648. Food and Drug Administration (HFI-35), 5600 Fishers Lane Rockville, MD 20857, USA.

[50] Swiderski, C.E. and French, D.D., "Paradigms for Parasite Control in Adult Horse Populations: A Review." *54th Annual Convention of the American Association of Equine Practitioners - AAEP*, 2008 - San Diego, CA, USA.

[51] Proudman CJ, French NP, Trees AJ. "Tapeworm infection is a significant risk factor for spasmodic colic and ileal impaction colic in the horse." *Equine Vet J* 1998; 30:194-199.

[52] L.E. Johnson, "The Parasite Puzzle: The Myths and Mysteries of Equine Parasitism," In: *NAVC Proceedings 2007, North American Veterinary Conference* (Eds). Publisher: NAVC (www.tnavc.org). Internet Publisher: International Veterinary Information Service, Ithaca NY (www.ivis.org), Last updated: 13-Jan-2007.

[53] *Merck Veterinary Manual*, Merck & Co., Inc.; New Jersey, 8 edition April 15, 1998. "Strongyloides sp."Horses: Tapeworms.

[54] Craig R. Reinemeyer, Douglas E. Hutchensb, 1, Wm. P. Eckbladc, 2, Alan A. Marchiondoc and Jack I. Shugartc "Dose-confirmation studies of the cestocidal activity of pyrantel pamoate paste in horses," *Veterinary Parasitology* Vol. 138, Issues 3-4, 15 June 2006, 234-239.

[55] Murray, M.J. *Ibid.*

[56] "Proglottids."

[57] Murray, M.J. *Ibid.*

[58] *Loc. cit.*

[59] *Loc. cit.*

[60] *Merck Veterinary Manual*, Merck & Co., Inc.; New Jersey, 8 edition April 15, 1998. "Strongyloides sp."Horses: Tapeworms.

[61] Murray, M.J. *Ibid.*

[62] *Loc. cit.*

[63] Craig R. Reinemeyer, Douglas E. Hutchens, Wm. P. Eckblad, Alan A. Marchiondo and Jack I. Shugart "Dose-confirmation studies of the cestocidal activity of pyrantel pamoate paste in horses," *Veterinary Parasitology* Vol. 138, Issues 3-4, 15 June 2006, 234-239.

[64] *Loc. cit.*

[65] Round, M.C., "Lungworm infection (*Dictyocaulus arnfieldi*) of horses and donkeys." *Vet Rec* 1976; 99:393-395; Matthews, J.B., "Parasitic Airway Disease." In: *Equine Respiratory Diseases*, Lekeux P. (Ed.) International Veterinary Information Service, Ithaca NY (www.ivis.org), 2002; B0327.0302 (Last Updated: 13-Mar-2002)

[66] Lyons ET, Tolliver SC, Drudge JH, *et al.* "Lungworms (*Dictyocaulus arnfieldi*): prevalence in live equids in Kentucky." *Am J Vet Res* (*American Journal of Veterinary Research*) 1985; 46:921-923.

[67] Matthews, J.B., "Parasitic Airway Disease." In: *Equine Respiratory Diseases*, Lekeux P. (Ed.) International Veterinary Information Service, Ithaca NY (www.ivis.org), 2002; B0327.0302 (Last Updated: 13-Mar-2002)

[68] *Loc. cit.*

[69] Jacobs DE. "Lungworm - *Dictocaulus arnfieldii*." In: *A Colour Atlas of Equine Parasites*. London: Balliere Tindall, 1986; 8.4-8.9.

[70] Round, M.C., "Lungworm infection (*Dictyocaulus arnfieldi*) of horses and donkeys." *Vet Rec* 1976; 99:393-395.

[71] Round MC. *A study of the natural history of lungworm infection of equidae*. PhD Thesis, University of Cambridge, 1972; Pandey VS. "Epidemiological observations on lungworm, *Dictyocaulus arnfieldi*, in donkeys from Morocco." *J Helminthol* (*Journal of Helminthology*) 1980; 54:275-279; Lyons ET, Tolliver SC, Drudge JH, *et al.* "Parasites in lungs of dead equids in Kentucky: emphasis on *Dictyocaulus arnfieldi*." *Am J Vet Res* 1985; 46:924-927.

[72] A. K. Thiemann and N. J. Bell, "The Peculiarities of Donkey Respiratory Disease." In: *Equine Respiratory Diseases*, Lekeux P. (Ed.) International Veterinary Information Service, Ithaca NY (www.ivis.org), 2001; B0330.1101 (Last Updated: 14-Nov-2001)

[73] Rose MA, Round MC, Beveridge WIB. "Influenza in horses and donkeys in Britain." *Vet Rec.* 1970; 86:768-769.

[74] Kubesy AA, Abdel-Hamid MA, El-Halim MMA *et al.* "The diagnostic value of transtracheal lavage. 1. Cytopathological and

parasitological findings of lavage fluids in some respiratory affections in equines." *Vet Med J Giza* 1991; 39(2):255-266; MacKay RJ, Urquhart KA. "An outbreak of eosinophilic bronchitis in horses possibly associated with *Dictyocaulus arnfieldi* infection." *Equine Vet J* 1979; 11:110-112.

[75] A. K. Thiemann and N. J. Bell, "The Peculiarities of Donkey Respiratory Disease." In: *Equine Respiratory Diseases*, Lekeux P. (Ed.) International Veterinary Information Service, Ithaca NY (www.ivis.org), 2001; B0330.1101 (Last Updated: 14-Nov-2001); see also Rode B, Jorgensen RJ. "Baermannization of Dictyocaulus spp. from faeces of cattle, sheep and donkeys." *Vet Parasitol* 1989; 30:205-211.

[76] Round MC. *A study of the natural history of lungworm infection of equidae.* PhD Thesis, University of Cambridge, 1972; MacKay RJ, Urquhart KA. "An outbreak of eosinophilic bronchitis in horses possibly associated with *Dictyocaulus arnfieldi* infection." *Equine Vet J* 1979; 11:110-112; Clayton HM, Trawford AF. "Anthelmintic control of lungworm in donkeys." *Equine Vet J* 1981; 13:192-194.

[77] Matthews, J.B., "Parasitic Airway Disease." In: *Equine Respiratory Diseases*, Lekeux P. (Ed.) International Veterinary Information Service, Ithaca NY (www.ivis.org), 2002; B0327.0302 (Last Updated: 13-Mar-2002)

[78] Kates KC, Colglazier ML, Enzie FD. "Oxibendazole: critical anthelmintic trials in equids." *Vet Rec* 1975; 97:442-444.

[79] Urch DL, Allen WR. "Studies on fenbendazole for treating lung and intestinal parasites in horses and donkeys." *Equine Vet J* 1980; 12:74-77.

[80] Clayton HM, Neave RM. "Efficacy of mebendazole against *Dictyocaulus arnfieldi* in the donkey." *Vet Rec* 1979; 104:571-572.

[81] Clayton HM, Trawford AF. "Anthelmintic control of lungworm in donkeys." *Equine Vet J* 1981; 13:192-194.

[82] Coles GC, Hillyer MH, Taylor FGR, *et al.* "Activity of moxidectin against bots and lungworm in equids." *Vet Rec* 1998; 143:169-170. See also Coles GC, Hillyer MH, Taylor FGR, Parker LD. "Activity of moxidectin against bots and lungworm in equids." *Vet Rec* 1998; 143(6):169-170.

[83] Britt DP, Preston JM. "Efficacy of ivermectin against *Dictyocaulus arnfieldi* in ponies." *Vet Rec* 1985; 116:343-345; Dixon PM, Railton DI, McGorum BC, *et al.* "Equine pulmonary disease: a case control study of 300 referred cases. Part 4: Treatments and re-examination findings." *Equine Vet J* 1995; 27:436-439.

[84] Reitsma JF. "The treatment of a lung worm infection in ponies with albendazole (Valbazen)." *Tijdschr Diergeneeskd* 1983; 108:569-571.

[85] A. K. Thiemann and N. J. Bell, "The Peculiarities of Donkey Respiratory Disease." In: *Equine Respiratory Diseases*, Lekeux P. (Ed.) International Veterinary Information Service, Ithaca NY (www.ivis.org), 2001; B0330.1101 (Last Updated: 14-Nov-2001)

[86] *Loc. Cit.*

[87] *Merck Veterinary Manual*, Merck & Co., Inc.; New Jersey, 8 edition April 15, 1998. "Strongyloides sp."TABLE 01: Recommended Treatments for Lungworms.

[88] S.R. Purdy, "Herd Health for Miniature Donkeys," In: *Veterinary Care of Donkeys*, Matthews N.S. and Taylor T.S. (Eds.). International Veterinary Information Service, Ithaca NY (www.ivis.org), Last updated: 1-Apr-2005; A2921.0405

[89] Payne, P.A., Carter, G.R., (Eds.). *A Concise Guide to the Microbial and Parasitic Diseases of Horses*, International Veterinary Information Service, Ithaca NY (www.ivis.org), Last updated: 30-Nov-2007; A4703.1107

[90] Swiderski CE. "Equine parasitic disease". In: Smith B, ed. *Large animal internal medicine*, 4th ed. St. Louis: Mosby Inc., 2008.; Swiderski, C.E. and French, D.D., "Paradigms for Parasite Control in Adult Horse Populations: A Review." *54th Annual Convention of the American Association of Equine Practitioners* - AAEP, 2008 - San Diego, CA, USA.

[91] *Merck Veterinary Manual*, Merck & Co., Inc.; New Jersey, 8 edition April 15, 1998. "Strongyloides sp."

[92] Code of Federal Regulations - Title 21: Food and Drugs (December 2005) 21 CFR 520.1195 - Ivermectin liquid. (USA)

[93] 21 CFR 520.1640 - Oxibendazole suspension.

Code of Federal Regulations - Title 21: Food and Drugs (December 2005) (USA).

[94] P. Nansen, S. Andersen and M. Hesselholt, "Experimental infection of the horse with Fasciola hepatica," *Experimental Parasitology* Volume 37, Issue 1, February 1975, 15-19.

[95] *Loc. cit.*

[96] Alves RM, van Rensburg LJ, van Wyk JA., "Fasciola in horses in the Republic of South Africa: a single natural case of Fasciola hepatica and the failure to infest ten horses either with F. hepatica or Fasciola gigantica." *Onderstepoort J Vet Res.* 1988 Sep;55(3):157-63.

[97] MA Valero, S Mas-Coma, "Comparative infectivity of Fasciola hepatica metacercariae from isolates of the main and secondary reservoir animal host species in the Bolivian Altiplano high human endemic region," *Folia Parasitologica* 47, 2000, 17-22.

[98] Owen J,M., "Liver fluke infection in horses and ponies," *Equine Vet J.* 1977 Jan;9(1):29-31.

[99] http://www.merckvetmanual.com/mvm/index.jsp?cfile=htm/bc/191505. htm&word=moxidectin

[100] Supplement to NADA 141-087 "5. Animal Safety
The approval of this supplemental NADA 141-087 is for a new indication. It does not change the dose level, frequency or route of administration of QUEST (moxidectin) 2% Equine Oral Gel or the class or species of treated animals. Consequently, no additional animal safety data were required for approval of this new indication. Information regarding the safety of QUEST Gel to treat horses and ponies is located in Section 5 (pages 19-27) of the original NADA 141-087 Freedom of Information Summary (July 11, 1997).
The precautions section of the labeling was modified in response to reports of misuse of the product in dogs."

[101] Study No. 0696-E-US-04-00

[102] *Loc. cit.*

[103] Boersema JH, Eysker M, van der Aar WM. "The reappearance of strongyle eggs in the faeces of horses after treatment with moxidectin." *Vet Q* (*Veterinary Quarterly*) 1998;20:12–15.

[104] von Samson-Himmelstjerna G, Fritzen B, Demeler J, *et al.* "Cases of reduced cyathostomin egg-reappearance period and failure of Parascaris equorum egg count reduction following ivermectin treatment as well as survey on pyrantel efficacy on German horse farms." *Vet Parasitol* 2007;144:74–80; Boersema JH, Eysker M, Maas J, *et al.* "Comparison of the reappearance of strongyle eggs on foals, yearlings and adult horses after treatment with ivermectin or pyrantel." *Vet Q* 1996;18:7–9.

[105] Eaton SA, Allen D, Eades SC, Schneider DA., "Digital Starling forces and hemodynamics during early laminitis induced by an aqueous extract of black walnut (Juglans nigra) in horses," *Am J Vet Res.* 1995 Oct; 56(10):1338-44; Galey, F.D. (University of California, Davis, CA); Twardock, A.R.; Goetz, T.E.; Schaeffer, D.J.; Hall, J.O.; Beasley, V.R., "Gamma scintigraphic analysis of the distribution of perfusion of blood in the equine foot during black walnut (Juglans nigra)-induced laminitis," *American Journal of Veterinary Research* (USA) April 1990, v. 51(4) p. 688-695.

[106] Bonkovsky, H.L., E.E. Cable, J.W. Cable, S.E. Donohue, E.C. White, Y.J. Greene, R.W. Lambrecht, K.K. Srivastava, W.N. Arnold, "Porphyrogenic properties of the terpenes camphor, pinene, and thujone (with a note on historic implications for absinthe and the illness of Vincent van Gogh)," *Biochem. Pharmacol.* 43:2359–2368, 1992; Jiří Patočka and Bohumil Plucar, "Pharmacology and toxicology of absinthe," *Journal of Applied Biomedicine* 1: 199–205, 2003.

[107] Patočka J. and B. Plucar, "Absint a jeho psychiatrická reflexe," *Psychiatrie* (2003) 7: 96–99.

[108] K.A. Tariq, ,M.Z. Chishti, F. Ahmad and A.S. Shawl, "Anthelmintic activity of extracts of Artemisia absinthium against ovine nematodes," *Veterinary Parasitology*, Vol. 160, Issues 1-2, 9 March 2009, 83-88.

[109] V. Beasley, "Toxicants that Cause Hemolysis," *Veterinary Toxicology*, Beasley V. (Ed.) International Veterinary Information Service, Ithaca NY (www.ivis.org), 1999; A2652.0899 Last Updated: 9-Aug-1999.

[110] Miyazawa K, Ito M, Ohsaki K., "An equine case of urticaria associated with dry garlic feeding," *J Vet Med Sci.* 1991 Aug;53

(4):747-8; Emanuela Valle, Barbara Padalino, "Garlic Effects In the Horse; A Clinical Report," Società Italiana Veterinari per Equini - SIVE - XII Congresso Multisala, Bologna, Italy 2006; Pearson, W., Boermans H.J., Betteger W.J., McBride B.W, Lindinger M.I., "Association of maximum voluntary dietary intake of freeze-dried garlic with Heinz body anemia in horses," *American Journal of Veterinary Research*, March 2005, Vol. 66, No. 3, 457-465; Rose P., Whiteman M., Moore P. K., Zhu Z.Y., Bioactive S- alk(en)yl cysteine sulfoxide metabolites in the genus Allium: the chemistry of potential therapeutic agents," *Nat. Prod. Rep.* (2005) 22, 351-368.

111 Lee KW, Yamato O, Tajima M, Kuraoka M, Omae S, Maede Y., "Hematologic changes associated with the appearance of eccentrocytes after intragastric administration of garlic extract to dogs," *Am J Vet Res.* 2000 Nov; 61(11):1446-50.

112 Pearson, W, Boermans, HJ, Bettger, WJ, McBride, BW, Lindinger, MI, "Safety assessment of freeze-dried garlic (Allium sativum) in horses: Heinz body anemia associated with maximum voluntary intake," *Am. J. Vet.* (2004) In Press; Wendy Pearson, Herman J. Boermans, William J. Bettger, Brian W. McBride,Michael I. Lindinger, "Association of maximum voluntary dietary intake of freeze-dried garlic with Heinz body anemia in horses," *American Journal of Veterinary Research,* March 2005, Vol. 66, No. 3, 457-465.

113 Qing Yang, Qiuhui Hub, Osamu Yamatoc, Keun-Woo Leed, Yoshimitsu Maedec, Teruhiko Yoshiharaa, "Organosulfur Compounds from Garlic (Allium sativum) Oxidizing Canine Erythrocytes," *Z. Naturforsch.* 58c, 408Ð412 (2003).

114 Pearson, W., "Ethnoveterinary Medicine: The Science of Botanicals in Equine Health and Disease," *Proceedings of the 2nd European Equine Health & Nutrition Congress*, (2003) Lelystad, The Netherlands, 31-40.

115 When rightly questioned on this by Victoria Ferguson, cf. http://www.herbalhorse.com/articles-pub/articles-index/garlic; W. Pearson, *per. litt.*

116 http://www.herbalhorse.com/articles-pub/articles-index/garlic

117 W. Pearson, *per. litt.*

118 Qing Yang, Qiuhui Hub, Osamu Yamatoc, Keun-Woo Leed, Yoshimitsu Maedec, Teruhiko Yoshiharaa, "Organosulfur Compounds from Garlic (Allium sativum) Oxidizing Canine Erythrocytes," *Z. Naturfors* 58c, 408Ð412 (2003).

119 Dixit, VP, Joshi, S, Sinha, R, Bharvava, SK, Varma, M., "Hypolipidemic activity of guggal resin (Commiphora mukul) and garlic (Alium sativum linn.) in dogs (Canis familiaris) and monkeys (Presbytis entellus entellus Dufresne)," *Biochem Exp Biol.* (1980) 16(4):421-4; Ronald T. Ackermann, MD; Cynthia D. Mulrow, MD, MSc; Gilbert Ramirez, DrPH; Christopher D. Gardner, PhD; Laura Morbidoni, MD; Valerie A. Lawrence, MD, MSc, "Garlic Shows Promise for Improving Some Cardiovascular Risk Factors," *Arch Intern Med.* (2001) 161:813-824.

120 Kurt M Reinhart, Craig I Coleman, Colleen Teevan, Payal Vachhani, C Michael White, "Effects of Garlic on Blood Pressure in Patients With and Without Systolic Hypertension: A Meta-Analysis," *The Annals of Pharmacotherapy*, (2008) Vol. 42, No. 12, pp. 1766-1771.

121 Carmia Borek, "Garlic Reduces Dementia and Heart-Disease Risk," *Supplement: Significance of Garlic and Its Constituents in Cancer and Cardiovascular Disease, American Society for Nutrition J. Nutr.* 136:810S-812S, March 2006.

122 In Dr Kellon's courses. See http://www.drkellon.com

123 http://gastrogard.us.merial.com/faq.asp; Dr Eleanor Kellon, *Per. Litt.*

124 A. P. Knight and R. G. Walter, *A Guide to Plant Poisoning of Animals in North America*, Knight A.P. and Walter R.G. (Eds.) Publisher: Teton New Media, Jackson WY (www.tetonnm.com/) Internet Publisher: International Veterinary Information Service, Ithaca NY (www.ivis.org), 2003; B0504.0403. Plants Affecting the Skin and Liver (Last Updated: 16-May-2003)

125 For example, tansy ragwort (*Senecio jacobaea*) is toxic to most animals (including humans), and is potentially lethal to cattle and horses, which can be poisoned by eating only 2-8% of their body weight. Its pyrrolizidine alkaloids cause hepatocellular necrosis, mitotic arrest and hepatic fibrosis. Signs of poisoning include central nervous signs, scouring, bloody droppings, rectal

prolapse, and weight loss, cf. Brent Hoff, Gary Thomson, Margaret Stalker, Robert Walsh, Kirsten Graham, Marcia R S Ilha, "Summer brings three 'herd outbreaks' of toxicities," *Animal Health Laboratory Newsletter*, University of Guelph Laboratory Services ,Volume 10, Number 3, September, 2006, 19; Tansy mustard has been associated with two different syndromes involving neurological symptoms, blindness, and aimless wandering in cattle, cf. A. P. Knight and R. G. Walter, "Plants Affecting the Skin and Liver (Part II)" in *A Guide to Plant Poisoning of Animals in North America*, Knight A.P. and Walter R.G. (Eds.) Publisher: Teton NewMedia, Jackson WY (www.veterinarywire.com) Internet Publisher: International Veterinary Information Service, Ithaca NY (www.ivis.org), 2003; B0504.0403 (Last Updated: 16-May-2003).

[126] TITLE 21--FOOD AND DRUGS: CHAPTER I--FOOD AND DRUG ADMINISTRATION DEPARTMENT OF HEALTH AND HUMAN SERVICES: SUBCHAPTER B--FOOD FOR HUMAN CONSUMPTION (CONTINUED) [Code of Federal Regulations] [Title 21, Volume 3] [Revised as of April 1, 2008] [CITE: 21CFR172.510] http://www.accessdata.fda.gov/scripts/cdrh/cfdocs/cfcfr/CFRSearch.cfm?fr=172.510

[127] Torald Sollmann, "Anthelmintics: Their Efficiency as Tested on Earthworms," *Journal of Pharmacology And Experimental Therapeutics*, Vol. 12, Issue 3, 129-170, 1918.

[128] *British Medical Journal*, 1947 August 9; 2(4518): 238.

[129] M.M. van Krimpen, G.P. Binnendijk, F. Borgsteede, C. Gaasenbeek, "In vivo testing of alternatives for conventional treatment of Ascaris suum in pigs," *Animal Sciences Group van Wageningen UR*, Rapport 82, November 2007, 17-21.

[130] *Loc. cit.*

[131] *Loc. cit.*

[132] KA Tariq, MZ Chishti, F Ahmad, AS Shawl, "Anthelmintic efficacy of Achillea millifolium against gastrointestinal nematodes of sheep: in vitro and in vivo studies," *Journal of Helminthology* (2008), 82:227-233 Cambridge University Press.

[133] Zafar Iqbal, Muhammad Lateef, Muhammad Shoaib Akhtar,

Muhammad Nabeel Ghayur and Anwarul Hassan Gilani, "In vivo anthelmintic activity of ginger against gastrointestinal nematodes of sheep," *Journal of Ethnopharmacology*, Volume 106, Issue 2, 30 June 2006, 285-287.

134 K.A. Tariq, M.Z. Chishti, F. Ahmad, A.S. Shawl and M.A. Tantray, "Evaluation of anthelmintic activity of Iris hookeriana against gastrointestinal nematodes of sheep," *Journal of Helminthology* (2008), 82:135-141 Cambridge University Press.

135 JM Burke, A Wells, P Casey, RM Kaplan, "Herbal dewormer fails to control gastrointestinal nematodes in goats," *Veterinary Parasitology,* 2008, Volume 160, Issues 1-2, 9 March 2009, 168-170.

136 JM Burke, A Wells, P Casey, JE Miller, "Garlic and papaya lack control over gastrointestinal nematodes in goats and lambs," *Veterinary Parasitology*, Volume 159, Issue 2, 5 February 2009, 171-174.

137 Satrija, F., Retnani, E.B., Ridwan, Y. and Tiuria, R., "Potential use of herbal anthelmintics as alternative antiparasitic drugs for small holder farms in developing countries," *Livestock Community and Environment. Proceedings of the 10th Conference of the Association of Institutions for Tropical Veterinary Medicine*, 2001, Copenhagen, Denmark.

138 *Loc.cit.*

139 Mursof, E. P. and He, S., "A potential role of papaya latex as an anthelmintic against patent Ascaridia galli infection in chickens," *Hemera Zoa*, 1991, 74:11-20.

140 Satrija, F., Nansen, P., Bjørn, H., Murtini, S. and He, S., "Effect of papaya latex (Carica papaya) against Ascaris suum in naturally infected pigs," *Journal of Helminthology*, 1994, 68: 343-346.

141 Satrija, F, "Anthelmintic activity of Indian mulberry fruit against Haemonchus contortus in sheep," Abstract 17th International Conference of WAAVP Copenhagen-Denmark (f.5.02), 1999.

142 Purwati, E., He, S., "Pengaruh getah papaya (Carica papaya) terhadap Ascaridia, galli dewasa in vitro," *Hemera Zoa*, 1991, 74: 6-10.

[143] Satrija, F., Nansen, P., Bjørn, H., Murtini, S., He, S., "Effect of papaya latex (Carica papaya) against Ascaris suum in naturally infected pigs," *Journal of Helminthology,* (1994) 68: 343-346.

[144] Satrija, F., P. Nansen, S. Murtini and He, S., "Anthelmintic activity of papaya latex against patent Heligmosomoides polygyrus infections in mice," *Journal of Ethnopharmacology*, (1995) 48: 161-164.

[145] Katz, H., "Desiccants: dry as dust means insect deaths," *Pest Control Technol.* (1991) April:82,'84; Abrams, H.K. "Diatomaceous earth pheumoconiosis," *Am. J. Public Health* (1954) 44-592-599.

[146] Insecticide. 61790-53-2. Accessed at http://www.fda.gov/downloads/Food/FoodSafety/FoodContaminantsAdulteration/Pesticides/ucm114655.pdf

[147] J. Hoyt Snyder, "Beyond Anthelmintics: Parasite Management in Small Ruminants," *NAVC Proceedings 2007, North American Veterinary Conference* (Eds). Publisher: NAVC (www.tnavc.org). Internet Publisher: International Veterinary Information Service, Ithaca NY (www.ivis.org), Last updated: 13-Jan-2007.

[148] H Checkoway, N J Heyer, P A Demers, N E Breslow, "Mortality among workers in the diatomaceous earth industry," *British Journal of Industrial Medicine* 1993;50:586-597; D. Post, "Low-risk Pest Management," *Clinical Avian Medicine,* Harrison G.J. and Lightfoot T.L. (Eds.). Publisher: Clinical Avian Medicine (www.clinicalavianmedicine.com). Internet Publisher: International Veterinary Information Service, Ithaca NY (www.ivis.org), Last updated: 19-Dec-2007; A3817.1207.

[149] Harvey Checkoway, Nicholas J. Heyer, Noah S. Seixas, Esther A. E. Welp, Paul A. Demers, Janet M. Hughes and Hans Weill, "Dose-Response Associations of Silica with Nonmalignant Respiratory Disease and Lung Cancer Mortality in the Diatomaceous Earth Industry," *American Journal of Epidemiology* Vol. 145, No. 8: 680-688.

[150] Celia M. Marr, "Weight Loss in the Adult Horse," *Proceedings of the 10th International Congress of World Equine Veterinary Association* 2008 - Moscow, Russia.

[151] C.R. Reinemeyer, "Controlling Strongyle Parasites of

Horses: A Mandate for Change," Proceedings of the 55th Annual Convention of the American Association of Equine Practitioners, 2009.

[152] L.E. Johnson, "The Parasite Puzzle: The Myths and Mysteries of Equine Parasitism," In: NAVC Proceedings 2007, North American Veterinary Conference (Eds). Publisher: NAVC (www.tnavc.org). Internet Publisher: International Veterinary Information Service, Ithaca NY (www.ivis.org), Last updated: 13-Jan-2007.

[153] C.R. Reinemeyer, "Controlling Strongyle Parasites of Horses: A Mandate for Change," *Proceedings of the 55th Annual Convention of the American Association of Equine Practitioners*, 2009.

[154] Proudman, CJ, French NP, Trees, AJ, "Tapeworm infection is a significant risk factor for spasmodic colic and ileal impaction colic in the horse," *Equine Vet J.* 1998; 30:194-199.

[155] Eysker M, Bakker J, van den Berg M, et al. The use of age-clustered pooled fecal samples for monitoring worm control in horses. *Vet Parasitol* 2008 151:249–255.

[156] NADA 120-648. Food and Drug Administration Freedom of Information Staff (HFI-35), 5600 Fishers Lane Rockville, MD 20857, USA.

[157] http://www.merckvetmanual.com/mvm/index.jsp?cfile=htm/bc/22505.htm

[158] Barger, I. A. "Benzimidazole resistance in small strongyle of horses," *Aust Vet J* (*Australian Veterinary Journal*) (1974), 55:594; French, D.D., Klei, T.R. "Benzimidazole resistant strongyle infections: a review of significance, occurrence, diagnosis, and control." In: *Proceedings of the 29th Annual American Association of Equine Practitioners Convention* (1983) 313; Dorny, P, Vercruysse J, Berghen P. "Resistance of small strongyles to benzimidazoles in Belgium." *J Vet Med* (*Journal of Veterinary Medicine*) Series B (1988) 35:72; Kaplan RM. "Anthelmintic resistance in nematodes of horses." *Vet Res* (2002) 33:491–507; Kaplan RM, Klei TR, Lyons ET, *et al.* "Prevalence of anthelmintic resistant cyathostomes on horse farms." *J Am Vet Med Assoc* 2004;225:903–910.

[159] Little, D., Flowers, J.R., Hammerberg, B.H., *et al.* "Management of drug-resistant cyathostomiosis on a breeding farm in central North Carolina." *Equine Vet J* (2004) 5:246; Drudge, J.H., Lyons, E.T. "Newer developments in helminth control and Strongylus vulgaris research." *Proceedings of the 11th Annual American Association of Equine Practitioners Convention.* 1965;378–383.

[160] P. Dorchies, "Anthelmintic Resistance and Control of Roundworms," *Proceedings of the 9th International Congress of World Equine Veterinary Association* 2006, Morocco.

[161] *Loc. cit.*

[162] von Samson-Himmelstjerna G, Fritzen B, Demeler J, *et al.* "Cases of reduced cyathostomin egg-reappearance period and failure of Parascaris equorum egg count reduction following ivermectin treatment as well as survey on pyrantel efficacy on German horse farms." *Vet Parasitol* 2007;144:74–80.

[163] Trawford A.F. and Burden F. "Ivermectin resistance in cyathostomes in four donkeys herds at the Donkey Sanctuary, UK." *Worldwide Association for the Advancement of Veterinary Parasitology*, Calgary, 2009.

[164] *Loc. cit.*

[165] Slocombe JOD, de Gannes RVG, Lake MC. "Macrocyclic lactone-resistant Parascaris equorum on stud farms in Canada and effectiveness of fenbendazole and pyrantel pamoate." *Vet Parasitol* 2007;145:371–376; Boersema JH, Eysker M, Nas JWM. "Apparent resistance of Parascaris equorum to macrocyclic lactones." *Vet Rec* 2002; 150:279–281; Craig TM, Diamond PL, Ferwerda NS, *et al.* "Evidence of ivermectin resistance by Parascaris equorum on a Texas horse farm." *J Equine Vet Sci* 2007;27:67–71; Hearn FP, Peregrine AS. "Identification of foals infected with Parascaris equorum apparently resistant to ivermectin." *J Am Vet Med Assoc* 2003;223:482–485; Schougaard H, Nielsen MK. "Apparent ivermectin resistance of Parascaris equorum in Danish foals." *Vet Rec* 2007;160:439–440.

[166] Bjorn, H., Sommer, C., Schougard, H., *et al.* "Resistance to benzimidazole anthelmintics in small strongyles (Cyathostominae) of horses in Denmark." *Acta Vet Scand* (*Acta Veterinaria Scandinavica*) (1991) 32:253.

[167] Kettle P. "Drenching policy can help breed resistant worms." *New Zeal J Agric* (*New Zealand Journal of Agriculture*) 1980;141:63; Webb R. "Epidemiological factors contributing to a high incidence of anthelmintic resistance in field populations in Haemonchus contortus." In: *Proceedings of the 2nd International Symposium on Veterinary Epidemiology and Economics* 1980;220–224.

[168] Personal conversations.

[169] Andrew S. Peregrine, "Deworming programs for horses: are we doing more harm than good?" *As Presented in the Rounds of Department of Large Animal Clinical Sciences Western College of Veterinary Medicine*, June/July 2005, Vol. 5, Issue 6.

[170] Swiderski, C.E. and French, D.D., "Paradigms for Parasite Control in Adult Horse Populations: A Review." *54th Annual Convention of the American Association of Equine Practitioners - AAEP*, 2008 - San Diego, CA, USA, citing: Michel JF. "Strategies for the use of anthelmintics in livestock and their implications for the development of drug resistance." *Parasitology* 1985;90:621–628.; Barnes EH, Dobson RJ. Population dynamics of Trichostrongylus columbriformis in sheep: computer model to stimulate grazing systems and the evaluation of anthelmintic resistance. *Int J Parasitol* (*International Journal of Parasitology*) 1990;20:823–831; Uhlinger C, Kristula M. "Effects of alternation of drug classes on the development of oxibendazole resistance in a herd of horses." *J Am Vet Med Assoc* 1992;201:51–55; Reinemeyer R, Henton JE. "Observations on equine strongyle control in southern temperate USA." *Equine Vet J* 1987;19:505–508; Little D, Flowers JR, Hammerberg BH, *et al*. "Management of drug-resistant cyathostominosis on a breeding farm in central North Carolina." *Equine Vet J* 2003;35:246–251.

[171] Swiderski, C.E. and French, D.D., "Paradigms for Parasite Control in Adult Horse Populations: A Review." *54th Annual Convention of the American Association of Equine Practitioners - AAEP*, 2008 - San Diego, CA, USA.

[172] Emily L. Brazik, Jan T. Luquire, Dianne Little, "Pyrantel pamoate resistance in horses receiving daily administration of pyrantel tartrate," *Journal of the American Veterinary Medical Association* (2006) 228:1, 101-103.

[173] J. Slocombe, M. Lake, "Efficacy of Daily Pyrantel Tartrate (Strongid C) against Strongyles in Ponies on Pasture," *Journal of Equine Veterinary Science*, Volume 27, Issue 10, Pages 439-445.

[174] *Loc.cit.*; Ray M. Kaplan, DVM, PhD, Thomas R. Klei, PhD Eugene T. Lyons, PhD, Guy Lester, DVM, PhD, Charles H. Courtney, DVM, PhD Dennis D. French, DVM, Sharon C. Tolliver, MS. N. Vidyashankar, PhD, Ying Zhao, MS, "Prevalence of anthelmintic resistant cyathostomes on horse farms," *Journal of the American Veterinary Medical Association*, September 15, 2004, Vol. 225, No. 6, 903-910.

[175] H. A. Brady, W. T. Nichols, M. Blanek and D. P. Hutcheson, "Parasite Resistance and the Effects of Rotational Deworming Regimens in Horses," In: *54th Annual Convention of the American Association of Equine Practitioners* - AAEP, 2008 - San Diego, CA, USA, (Ed.). Publisher: American Association of Equine Practitioners, Orlando, FL. Internet Publisher: International Veterinary Information Service, Ithaca NY (www.ivis.org), Last updated: 10-Dec-2008; P11173.1208.

[176] H. A. Brady, W. T. Nichols, M. Blanek and D. P. Hutcheson, "Parasite Resistance and the Effects of Rotational Deworming Regimens in Horses," In: *54th Annual Convention of the American Association of Equine Practitioners* - AAEP, 2008 - San Diego, CA, USA, (Ed.). Publisher: American Association of Equine Practitioners, Orlando, FL. Internet Publisher: International Veterinary Information Service, Ithaca NY (www.ivis.org), Last updated: 10-Dec-2008; P11173.1208.

[177] C.R. Reinemeyer, "Controlling Strongyle Parasites of Horses: A Mandate for Change," *Proceedings of the 55th Annual Convention of the American Association of Equine Practitioners*, 2009.

[178] *Loc. cit.*

[179] Herd RP. "Epidemiology and control of equine strongylosis at Newmarket." *Equine Vet J* 1986;18:447–452.

[180] Helle O, Velle W, Tharaldsen J. "Effect of ovine urine and some of its components on viability of nematode eggs and larvae in sheep faeces." *Vet Parasitol* 1989;32:349–354.

[181] C.R. Reinemeyer, "Controlling Strongyle Parasites of

Horses: A Mandate for Change," *Proceedings of the 55th Annual Convention of the American Association of Equine Practitioners*, 2009.

[182] Abamectin, ivermectin, eprinomectin, doramectin kill flies and dung beetles in the manure, cf. Holter. P., L. Strong, R. Wall, K. Wardhaugh, R. Herd. 1994, "Effects of ivermectin on pastureland ecology," *Veterinary Record* 135:211-212; Floate, K. D., "Off-target effects of ivermectin on insects and on dung degradation in southern Alberta, Canada," *Bull. Entomol. Res.* (1998) 88:25-35; Fincher, G. T., "Injectable ivermectin for cattle: Effects on some dung-inhabiting insects," *Environ. Entomol.* (1992) 21: 871-876.

Moxidectin is far less toxic to dung beetles and did not reduce dung beetle survival, cf. *Loc.cit.*; Lumaret, J. P. and F. Errouissi, "Use of anthelmintics in herbivores and evaluation of risks for the non target fauna of pastures," *Vet. Res.* (2002) 33: 547-562.

[183] Pamela Kay Wilson – 2005 Churchill Fellow, "Improving the Selection of Foreign Dung Beetle Species and Enhancing their Populations in Australia by Comparing the Effects of Grazing Activities in Natural and Transformed South African Environments," The Winston Churchill Memorial Trust of Australia, at http://www.dungbeetles.com.au/files/ChurchillTrustFinal.pdf

[184] The numbers of strongyle larvae available on pasture roughs were 15 times greater than on pasture lawns.
Herd RP, Willardson KL. "Seasonal distribution of infective strongyle larvae on horse pastures." *Equine Vet J* 1985;17: 235–237.

[185] Parnell IW. "Note on the survival of the eggs and free-living larvae of sclerostomes on pasture." *Scientific Agriculture* 1936;16:391–397.

[186] Ogbourne CP. "Pathogenesis of cyathostome (Trichonema) infection of the horse. A review." *Inst. Helmint.*, Comm. Agric. Bureaux, Farnham Royal Slough. Miscellaneous Publication no 5, 1978;1–25; Reinemeyer CR. "Small strongyles. Recent advances." *Vet Clin North Am Equine Pract* 1986;2:281–312.

[187] Swiderski, C.E. and French, D.D., "Paradigms for Parasite Control in Adult Horse Populations: A Review." *54th Annual Convention of the American Association of Equine Practitioners* - AAEP, 2008 - San Diego, CA, USA.

[188] Herd RP, Willardson KL, Gabel AA. "Epidemiological approach to the control of horse strongyles." *Equine Vet J* 1985; 17:202–207.

[189] Nielsen MK, Kaplan RM, Thamsborg SM, *et al.* "Climatic influences on development and survival of free-living stages of equine strongyles: implications for worm control strategies and managing anthelmintic resistance." *Vet J* 2007; 174:23–32; Baudena MA, Chapman MR, French DD, *et al.* "Seasonal development and survival of equine cyathostome larvae on pasture in south Louisiana." *Vet Parasitol* 2000;88:51–60.

[190] Reinemeyer CR. "Small strongyles. Recent advances." *Vet Clin North Am Equine Pract.* 1986 Aug;2(2):281-312.

[191] Nielsen MK, Kaplan RM, Thamsborg SM, *et al.* Climatic influences on development and survival of free-living stages of equine strongyles: implications for worm control strategies and managing anthelmintic resistance. *Vet J* 2007; 174:23–32; Kuzmina TA, Kuzmin YI, Kharchenko VA. "Field study on the survival, migration and overwintering of infective larvae of horse strongyles on pasture in central Ukraine." *Vet Parasitol* 2006;141:264–272.

[192] *Loc. cit.*; Reinemeyer CR. "Small strongyles. Recent advances." *Vet Clin North Am Equine Pract.* 1986 Aug;2 (2) :281-312.

[193] Reinemeyer C.R. "Controlling Strongyle Parasites of Horses: A Mandate for Change," *Proceedings of the 55th Annual Convention of the American Association of Equine Practitioners,* 2009.

[194] Rolfe PF, Dawson KL, Holm-Martin M. "Efficacy of moxidectin and other anthelmintics against small strongyles in horses." *Aust Vet J* 1998;76:332–334;

[195] Swiderski, C.E. and French, D.D., "Paradigms for Parasite Control in Adult Horse Populations: A Review." *54th Annual Convention of the American Association of Equine Practitioners* - AAEP, 2008 - San Diego, CA, USA.

[196] C.R. Reinemeyer, "Controlling Strongyle Parasites of Horses: A Mandate for Change," *Proceedings of the 55th Annual Convention of the American Association of Equine Practitioners,* 2009.

197 *Loc. cit.*

198 Boersema JH, Eysker M, Maas J, *et al.* "Comparison of the reappearance of strongyle eggs on foals, yearlings and adult horses after treatment with ivermectin or pyrantel." *Vet Q* 1996;18:7–9; von Samson-Himmelstjerna G, Fritzen B, Demeler J, *et al.* "Cases of reduced cyathostomin egg-reappearance period and failure of Parascaris equorum egg count reduction following ivermectin treatment as well as survey on pyrantel efficacy on German horse farms." *Vet Parasitol* 2007;144:74–80. However, Reinemeyer lists the ERP for Pyrantel pamoate as 4 weeks. Reinemeyer, C.R. "Controlling Strongyle Parasites of Horses: A Mandate for Change," *Proceedings of the 55th Annual Convention of the American Association of Equine Practitioners*, 2009.

199 Little D, Flowers JR, Hammerberg BH, *et al.* "Management of drug-resistant cyathostominosis on a breeding farm in central North Carolina." *Equine Vet J* 2003;35:246–251; von Samson-Himmelstjerna G, Fritzen B, Demeler J, *et al.* "Cases of reduced cyathostomin egg-reappearance period and failure of Parascaris equorum egg count reduction following ivermectin treatment as well as survey on pyrantel efficacy on German horse farms." *Vet Parasitol* 2007;144:74–80; Mercier P, Chick B, Alves-Branco F, *et al.* "Comparative efficacy, persistent effect, and treatment intervals of anthelmintic pastes in naturally infected horses." *Vet Parasitol* 2001;99:29–39.

200 Lind EO, Kuzmina T, Uggla A, *et al.* "A field study on the effect of some anthelmintics on cyathostomins of horses in Sweden." *Vet Res Commun* (*Veterinary Research Communications*) 2007;31:53–65; Boersema JH, Eysker M, van der Aar WM. "The reappearance of strongyle eggs in the faeces of horses after treatment with moxidectin." *Vet Q* 1998;20:12–15; Boersema JH, Eysker M, Maas J, *et al.* "Comparison of the reappearance of strongyle eggs on foals, yearlings and adult horses after treatment with ivermectin or pyrantel." *Vet Q* 1996;18:7–9; von Samson-Himmelstjerna G, Fritzen B, Demeler J, *et al.* "Cases of reduced cyathostomin egg-reappearance period and failure of Parascaris equorum egg count reduction following ivermectin treatment as well as survey on pyrantel efficacy on German horse farms." *Vet Parasitol* 2007;144:74–80.

[201] Boersema JH, Eysker M, van der Aar WM. "The reappearance of strongyle eggs in the faeces of horses after treatment with moxidectin." *Vet Q* 1998;20:12–15.

[202] Reinemeyer C.R. "Controlling Strongyle Parasites of Horses: A Mandate for Change," *Proceedings of the 55th Annual Convention of the American Association of Equine Practitioners*, 2009.

[203] Swiderski, C.E. and French, D.D., "Paradigms for Parasite Control in Adult Horse Populations: A Review." *54th Annual Convention of the American Association of Equine Practitioners* - AAEP, 2008 - San Diego, CA, USA.

[204] *Loc. cit.*

[205] Eysker M, Bakker J, van den Berg M, *et al.* "The use of age-clustered pooled fecal samples for monitoring worm control in horses." *Vet Parasitol* 2008 151:249–255; Gomez HH, Georgi JR. "Equine helminth infections: control by selective chemotherapy." *Equine Vet J* 1991;23:198– 200; Matthee S, McGeoch MA. "Helminths in horses: use of selective treatment for the control of strongyles." *J S Afr Vet Assoc* (*Journal of the South African Veterinary Association*) 2004;75:129–136; Duncan JL, Love S. "Preliminary observations on an alternative strategy for the control of horse strongyles." *Equine Vet J* 1991;23:226–228; Krecek RC, Guthrie AJ, Nieuwenhuizen LV, *et al.* "A comparison between the effects of conventional and selective antiparasitic treatments on nematode parasites of horses from two management schemes." *J S Afr Vet Assoc* 1994;65: 97–100.

[206] Reinemeyer C.R. "Controlling Strongyle Parasites of Horses: A Mandate for Change," *Proceedings of the 55th Annual Convention of the American Association of Equine Practitioners*, 2009.

[207] *Loc. cit.*

[208] Charts inlfuenced by Reinemeyer, *Loc.cit.*

[209] This is a guide only. Please read individual labeling. Be aware that product names also change from time to time.

Bibliography

Abrams, H.K. "Diatomaceous earth pheumoconiosis," *Am. J. Public Health* (1954) 44-592-599.

Ackermann, R.T.,MD; Cynthia D. Mulrow, MD, MSc; Gilbert Ramirez, DrPH; Christopher D. Gardner, PhD; Laura Morbidoni, MD. V.A. Lawrence, MD, MSc, "Garlic Shows Promise for Improving Some Cardiovascular Risk Factors," *Arch Intern Med.* (2001) 161:813-824.

Alves RM, van Rensburg LJ, van Wyk JA., "Fasciola in horses in the Republic of South Africa: a single natural case of Fasciola hepatica and the failure to infest ten horses either with F. hepatica or Fasciola gigantica." *Onderstepoort J Vet Res.* 1988 Sep;55(3):157-63.

Azevedo, J., P. R. Stout, "Farm Animal Manures: an Overview of their Role in the Agricultural Environment," *Univ. Of CA College of Agriculture Manual* 44 (1974).

Barger, I. A. "Benzimidazole resistance in small strongyle of horses," *Aust Vet J* (1974), 55:594; French, D.D., Klei, T.R. "Benzimidazole resistant strongyle infections: a review of significance, occurrence, diagnosis, and control." In: *Proceedings of the 29th Annual American Association of Equine Practitioners Convention* (1983) 313.

Barnes EH, Dobson RJ. "Population dynamics of Trichostrongylus columbriformis in sheep: computer model to stimulate grazing systems and the evaluation of anthelmintic resistance." *Int J Parasitol* 1990;20:823–831.

Bary, A.I., CG Cogger, DM Sullivan, *Fertilizing with manure.* A Pacific Northwest Extension Publication, Washington, Oregon, Idaho, July 2004. PNW0533. 1.

Baudena, MA, Chapman, MR, Horohov, DW, *et al.* "Protective responses against cyathostome infections." *Proceedings of the 19th International WAAVP Conference*, 2003.

Bjorn, H., Sommer, C., Schougard, H., *et al.* "Resistance to benzimidazole anthelmintics in small strongyles (Cyathostominae) of horses in Denmark." *Acta Vet Scand* (1991) 32:253.

Boersema JH, Borgsteede FHM, Eysker M, Elema TE, Gaasenbeek CPH and Burg van der WPJ, "The prevalence of anthelmintic resistance of horse strongyles in the Netherlands," *Vet. Quart.* (*Veterinary Quarterly*) 1991

Boersema JH, Eysker M, Maas J and Aar van der WM, "Comparison of the reappearance of strongyle eggs in foals, yearlings, and adult horses after treatment with ivermectin or pyrantel," *Vet. Quart.* 1996

Boersema JH, Eysker M, van der Aar WM. "The reappearance of strongyle eggs in the faeces of horses after treatment with moxidectin." *Vet. Quart.* 1998; 20:12–15.

Boersema JH, Eysker M, Nas JWM. "Apparent resistance of Parascaris equorum to macrocyclic lactones." *Vet Rec* 2002; 150:279–281.

Bonkovsky H.L., E.E. Cable, J.W. Cable, S.E. Donohue, E.C. White, Y.J. Greene, R.W. Lambrecht, K.K. Srivastava, W.N. Arnold, "Porphyrogenic properties of the terpenes camphor, pinene, and thujone (with a note on historic implications for absinthe and the illness of Vincent van Gogh)," *Biochem. Pharmacol.* 43:2359–2368, 1992.

Borek, C., "Garlic Reduces Dementia and Heart-Disease Risk," *Supplement: Significance of Garlic and Its Constituents in Cancer and Cardiovascular Disease*, American Society for Nutrition *J. Nutr.* 136:810S-812S, March 2006.

Brady H. A., W. T. Nichols, M. Blanek and D. P. Hutcheson, "Parasite Resistance and the Effects of Rotational Deworming Regimens in Horses," In: *54th Annual Convention of the American Association of Equine Practitioners* - AAEP, 2008 - San Diego, CA, USA, (Ed.). Publisher: American Association of Equine Practitioners, Orlando, FL. Internet Publisher: International Veterinary Information Service, Ithaca NY (www.ivis.org), Last updated: 10-Dec-2008; P11173.1208.

Brazik, E.L., Jan T. Luquire, Dianne Little, "Pyrantel pamoate resistance in horses receiving daily administration of pyrantel tartrate," *Journal of the American Veterinary Medical Association* (2006) 228:1, 101-103.

Britt DP, Preston JM. Efficacy of ivermectin against *Dictyocaulus arnfieldi* in ponies. *Vet Rec* 1985; 116:343-345

Burke, J.M., A Wells, P Casey, RM Kaplan, "Herbal dewormer fails to control gastrointestinal nematodes in goats," *Veterinary Parasitology*, 2008, Volume 160, Issues 1-2, 9 March 2009, 168-170.

Burke, J.M., A Wells, P Casey, JE Miller, "Garlic and papaya lack control over gastrointestinal nematodes in goats and lambs," *Veterinary Parasitology*, Volume 159, Issue 2, 5 February 2009, 171-174.

Checkoway, H., N. J. Heyer, P A Demers, N E Breslow, "Mortality among workers in the diatomaceous earth industry," *British Journal of Industrial Medicine* 1993;50:586-597.

Checkoway, H., Nicholas J. Heyer, Noah S. Seixas, Esther A. E. Welp, Paul A. Demers, Janet M. Hughes and Hans Weill, "Dose-Response Associations of Silica with Nonmalignant Respiratory Disease and Lung Cancer Mortality in the Diatomaceous Earth Industry," *American Journal of Epidemiology* Vol. 145, No. 8: 680-688.

Clayton HM, Neave RM. "Efficacy of mebendazole against *Dictyocaulus arnfieldi* in the donkey." *Vet Rec* 1979; 104:571-572.

Clayton HM, Trawford AF. "Anthelmintic control of lungworm in donkeys." *Equine Vet J* 1981; 13:192-194.

Coles GC, Hillyer MH, Taylor FGR, *et al*. "Activity of moxidectin against bots and lungworm in equids." *Vet Rec* 1998; 143:169-170.

Coles GC, Jackson F, Pomroy WE, *et al*. "The detection of anthelmintic resistance in nematodes of veterinary importance." *Vet Parasitol* 2006;136:167–185.

Combs, D. K., R. D. Goodrich, T. S. Kahlon and J. C.Meiske, "Effects of nonnutritional sources of variation on concentrations of various minerals in cattle hair," *Minnesota Cattle Feeders Rep*. (1979) 54.

Anne Couroucé-Malblanc, G. Fortier, M. Moulin, J, J.P. Valette, L. Petit, S. Dumontier, P.H. Pitel, "Reference Values on Hematologic and Biochemical Parameters in French Donkeys," *Proceedings of the 10th International Congress of World Equine Veterinary Association.* 2008 - Moscow, Russia.

Craig TM, Diamond PL, Ferwerda NS, *et al*. "Evidence of ivermectin resistance by Parascaris equorum on a Texas horse farm." *J Equine Vet Sci* 2007;27:67–71.

DiPietro, J.A., DVM, MS; Thomas Klei, PhD; and Craig Reinemeyer, DVM, PhD, "Efficacy of Fenbendazole Against Encysted Small Strongyle Larvae," *Proceedings of the Annual Convention of the AAEP*, 1997, 343-344.

Dixit V.P., Joshi S, Sinha R, Bharvava SK, Varma M., "Hypolipidemic activity of guggal resin (Commiphora mukul) and garlic (Alium sativum linn.) in dogs (Canis familiaris) and monkeys (Presbytis entellus entellus Dufresne)," *Biochem Exp Biol.* (1980) 16(4):421-4.

Dixon PM, Railton DI, McGorum BC, *et al.* "Equine pulmonary disease: a case control study of 300 referred cases. Part 4: Treatments and re-examination findings." *Equine Vet J* 1995;

Dopfer D, Kerssens CM, Meijer YG, *et al.* "Shedding consistency of strongyle-type eggs in Dutch boarding horses." *Vet Parasitol* 2004;124:249–258.

Dorchies, P., "Anthelmintic Resistance and Control of Roundworms," *Proceedings of the 9th International Congress of World Equine Veterinary Association* 2006, Morocco.

Dorny, P, Vercruysse J, Berghen P. "Resistance of small strongyles to benzimidazoles in Belgium." *J Vet Med Series B* (1988) 35:72;

Drudge, J.H., Lyons, E.T. "Newer developments in helminth control and Strongylus vulgaris research." *Proceedings of the 11th Annual American Association of Equine Practitioners Convention.* 1965;378–383.

Drudge JH, Lyons ET. "Control of internal parasites of the horse." *J Am Vet Med Assoc* 1966;148:378-383.

Duncan, J.L., Pirie HM., "The life cycle of Strongylus vulgaris in the horse," *Res Vet Sci.* (1972) Jul;13(4):374-9.

Duncan JL, Love S. "Preliminary observations on an alternative strategy for the control of horse strongyles." *Equine Vet J* 1991;23:226–228.

Eaton SA, Allen D, Eades SC, Schneider DA., "Digital Starling forces and hemodynamics during early laminitis induced by an aqueous extract of black walnut (Juglans nigra) in horses," *Am J Vet Res.* 1995 Oct; 56(10):1338-44.

Eysker M, Bakker J, van den Berg M, *et al.* "The use of age-clustered pooled fecal samples for monitoring worm control in horses." *Vet Parasitol* (2008) 151:249–255.

Fincher, G. T., "Injectable ivermectin for cattle: Effects on some dung-inhabiting insects," *Environ. Entomol.* (1992) 21: 871-876.

Fincher, G. T. and G. T. Wang, "Injectable moxidectin for cattle-Effects on 2 species of dung burying beetles (Coleoptera, Scarabaeidae)," *Southwest. Entomol.* (1992) 17:303-306.

Floate, K. D., "Off-target effects of ivermectin on insects and on dung degradation in southern Alberta, Canada," *Bull. Entomol. Res.* (1998) 88:25-35.

Fougère Barbara J; Susan G Wynn, *Veterinary Herbal Medicine*, St. Louis : Mosby, an affiliate of Elsevier, 2007.

Galey, F.D. (University of California, Davis, CA); Twardock, A.R.; Goetz, T.E.; Schaeffer, D.J.; Hall, J.O.; Beasley, V.R., "Gamma scintigraphic analysis of the distribution of perfusion of blood in the equine foot during black walnut (Juglans nigra)-induced laminitis," *American Journal of Veterinary Research* (USA) April 1990, v. 51(4) p. 688-695.

Giles, C.J., Urquhart KA, Longstaffe J, "Larval cyathostomosiasis (immature trichostronema-induced enteropathy): a report of 15 clinical cases," *Equine Veterinary Journal* 1985;17:196–201.

Godwin, D. and J, A. Moore, *Manure Management in Small Farm Livestock Operations, Protecting Surface and Groundwater*. EM8649 (Oregon State University, Cooperative Extension Service, 1997).

Gomez HH, Georgi JR. "Equine helminth infections: control by selective chemotherapy." *Equine Vet J 1991*;23:198–200.

Hayes, W.J. and E.R. Laws (eds.). 1990. *Handbook of Pesticide Toxicology, Classes of Pesticides*, Vol. 3. Academic Press, Inc., NY.

Hearn F.P.D, Peregrine A.S., "Identification of foals infected with Parascaris equorum apparently resistant to ivermectin." *JAVMA* (*Journal of the American Veterinary Medical Association*) 2003; 223: 482-85.

Helle O, Velle W, Tharaldsen J. "Effect of ovine urine and some of its components on viability of nematode eggs and larvae in sheep faeces." *Vet Parasitol* 1989;32:349–354.

Herd RP. "Epidemiology and control of equine strongylosis at Newmarket." *Equine Vet J* 1986;18:447–452.

Noritaka Hirazawa, Taro Ohtaka and Kazuhiko Hata, "Challenge trials on the anthelmintic effect of drugs and natural agents against the monogenean Heterobothrium okamotoi in the tiger puffer Takifugu rubripes." *Aquaculture*, Volume 188, Issues 1-2, 1 August 2000, 1-13.

Hodgkinson Jane E., "Cyathostomosis: Epidemiology and control," *Proceedings of the 47th British Equine Veterinary Association Congress* 2008.

Hoff, B., Gary Thomson, Margaret Stalker, Robert Walsh, Kirsten Graham, Marcia R S Ilha, "Summer brings three 'herd outbreaks' of toxicities," *Animal Health Laboratory Newsletter*, University of Guelph Laboratory Services ,Volume 10, Number 3, September, 2006, 19.

Holter, P., L. Strong, R. Wall, K. Wardhaugh, R. Herd, "Effects of ivermectin on pastureland ecology," *Veterinary Record* (1994) 135:211-212.

Hoyt Snyder, J. "Beyond Anthelmintics: Parasite Management in Small Ruminants," *NAVC Proceedings 2007, North American Veterinary Conference* (Eds). Publisher: NAVC (www.tnavc.org). Internet Publisher: International Veterinary Information Service, Ithaca NY (www.ivis.org), Last updated: 13-Jan-2007.

Iqbal, Z., Muhammad Lateef, Muhammad Shoaib Akhtar, Muhammad Nabeel Ghayur and Anwarul Hassan Gilani, "In vivo anthelmintic activity of ginger against gastrointestinal nematodes of sheep," *Journal of Ethnopharmacology*, Volume 106, Issue 2, 30 June 2006, 285-287.

Jenkins, J. *The Humanure Handbook*, Jenkins Publishing, Pennsylvania, 2nd ed, 1999.

Johnson L.E., "The Parasite Puzzle: The Myths and Mysteries of Equine Parasitism," In: *NAVC Proceedings 2007, North American Veterinary Conference* (Eds). Publisher: NAVC (www.tnavc.org). Internet Publisher: International Veterinary Information Service, Ithaca NY (www.ivis.org), Last updated: 13-Jan-2007.

Kaplan RM., "Anthelmintic resistance in nematodes of horses," *Vet Res* (*Veterinary Research*) 2002;33

Kaplan, R.M. DVM, PhD, Thomas R. Klei, PhD Eugene T. Lyons, PhD, Guy Lester, DVM, PhD, Charles H. Courtney, DVM, PhD Dennis D. French, DVM, Sharon C. Tolliver, MS. N. Vidyashankar, PhD, Ying Zhao, MS "Prevalence of anthelmintic resistant cyathostomes on horse farms," *Journal of the American Veterinary Medical Association*, September 15, 2004, Vol. 225, No. 6, 903-910.

Kates KC, Colglazier ML, Enzie FD. "Oxibendazole: critical anthelmintic trials in equids." *Vet Rec* 1975; 97:442-444.

Katz, H. 1991, "Desiccants: dry as dust means insect deaths," *Pest Control Technol.* April:82, 84.

Kettle P. "Drenching policy can help breed resistant worms." *New Zeal J Agric* 1980;141:63.

King, C. BVSc, MACVSc, MVetClinStud, *Natural Dewormers*, at http://www.animavet.com/NaturalDewormers.pdf

Kirchgessner M, Grassman E. *The dynamics of copper absorption.* In: Mills CF, ed. *Trace element metabolism in animals*. Edinburgh: Livingston, 1970:277–87.

Krecek RC, Guthrie AJ, Nieuwenhuizen LV, *et al.* "A comparison between the effects of conventional and selective antiparasitic treatments on nematode parasites of horses from two management schemes." *J S Afr Vet Assoc* 1994;65: 97–100.

Kubesy AA, Abdel-Hamid MA, El-Halim MMA *et al.* "The diagnostic value of transtracheal lavage. 1. Cytopathological and parasitological findings of lavage fluids in some respiratory affections in equines." *Vet Med J Giza* 1991; 39(2):255-266.

Kuzmina TA, Kuzmin YI, Kharchenko VA. "Field study on the survival, migration and overwintering of infective larvae of horse strongyles on pasture in central Ukraine." *Vet Parasitol* 2006;141:264–272.

Lankas, G.R and L.R. Gordon. Toxicology in W.C. Campbell (ed.). 1989. "Ivermectin and Abamectin." Springer-Verlag, NY.

Lee, K.W., Yamato O, Tajima M, Kuraoka M, Omae S, Maede Y., "Hematologic changes associated with the appearance of eccentrocytes after intragastric administration of garlic extract to dogs," *Am J Vet Res.* 2000 Nov; 61(11):1446-50.

Matthee S, McGeoch MA. "Helminths in horses: use of selective treatment for the control of strongyles." *J S Afr Vet Assoc* 2004;75:129–136.

Mercier P, Chick B, Alves-Branco F, *et al.* "Comparative efficacy, persistent effect, and treatment intervals of anthelmintic pastes in naturally infected horses." *Vet Parasitol* 2001;99:29–39.

Lind EO, Kuzmina T, Uggla A, *et al.* "A field study on the effect of some anthelmintics on cyathostomins of horses in Sweden." *Vet Res Commun* 2007;31:53–65

Lindgrena, K., Ö. Ljungvallb, O. Nilssonc, B.-L. Ljungströmd, C. Lindahla and J. Höglund, "Parascaris equorum in foals and in their environment on a Swedish stud farm, with notes on treatment failure of ivermectin," *Veterinary Parasitology*, Volume 151, Issues 2-4, 14 February 2008, 337-343.

Little, D., Flowers, J.R., Hammerberg, B.H., *et al.* "Management of drug-resistant cyathostomiosis on a breeding farm in central North Carolina." *Equine Vet J* (2004) 5:246-251.

Love, S., Murphy D, Mellor D, "Pathogenicity of cyathostome infection," *Vet Parasitol* (1999) 85:113-121.

Lumaret, J. P. and F. Errouissi, "Use of anthelmintics in herbivores and evaluation of risks for the non target fauna of pastures," *Vet. Res.* (2002) 33: 547-562.

Lyons ET, Tolliver SC, Drudge JH, *et al.* "Lungworms (*Dictyocaulus arnfieldi*): prevalence in live equids in Kentucky." *Am J Vet Res* (*American Journal of Veterinary Research*) 1985; 46:921-923.

McCraw, B.M. and J. O. D. Slocombe, "Early Development of and Pathology Associated with Strongylus edentatus," *Can J Comp Med.* 1974 April; 38(2): 124–138.

McCraw, B.M. and J O Slocombe, "Strongylus equinus: development and pathological effects in the equine host," *Can J Comp Med.* 1985 October; 49(4): 372–383.

MacKay RJ, Urquhart KA. "An outbreak of eosinophilic bronchitis in horses possibly associated with *Dictyocaulus arnfieldi* infection." *Equine Vet J* 1979; 11:110-112.

Marr Celia M, "Weight Loss in the Adult Horse," *Proceedings of the 10th International Congress of World Equine Veterinary Association* 2008 - Moscow, Russia.

Matthews, J.B., "Parasitic Airway Disease." In: *Equine Respiratory Diseases*, Lekeux P. (Ed.) International Veterinary Information Service, Ithaca NY (www.ivis.org), 2002; B0327.0302 (Last Updated: 13-Mar-2002)

Merck Veterinary Manual, Merck & Co., Inc.; New Jersey, 8 edition April 15, 1998.

Michel JF. "Strategies for the use of anthelmintics in livestock and their implications for the development of drug resistance." *Parasitology* 1985;90:621–628.

Miyazawa, K., Ito, M., Ohsaki, K., "An equine case of urticaria associated with dry garlic feeding," *J Vet Med Sci.* 1991 Aug;53(4):747-8.

Monahan C., "Anthelmintic Control Strategies for Horses," in *Companion and Exotic Animal Parasitology*, Bowman D.D. (Ed.), International Veterinary Information Service, Ithaca NY 2000; A0309.0500.

Murray, M.J., "Treatment of Equine Gastrointestinal Parasites," *8th Congress on Equine Medicine and Surgery,* 2003 - Geneva, Switzerland, Chuit P., Kuffer A. and Montavon S. (Eds.) International Veterinary Information Service, Ithaca, NY.

Mursof, E. P., He, S., "A potential role of papaya latex as an anthelmintic against patent Ascaridia galli infection in chickens," *Hemera Zoa*, 1991, 74:11-20.

NADA 120-648. Food and Drug Administration (HFI-35), 5600 Fishers Lane Rockville, MD 20857, USA.

Nadeau, J. "How to Properly Manage Manure," *Department of Animal Science Extension Articles*, University of Connecticut, 2006.

Nansen P., S. Andersen and M. Hesselholt, "Experimental infection of the horse with Fasciola hepatica," *Experimental Parasitology* Volume 37, Issue 1, February 1975, 15-19.

Nielsen MK, Haaning N, Olsen SN. "Strongyle egg shedding consistency in horses on farms using selective therapy in Denmark." *Vet Parasitol* 2006;135:333–335.

Nielsen MK, Kaplan RM, Thamsborg SM, *et al*. "Climatic influences on development and survival of free-living stages of equine strongyles: implications for worm control strategies and managing anthelmintic resistance." *Vet J* 2007; 174:23–32.

Ogbourne CP. "Observations on the free-living stages of strongylid nematodes of the horse." *Parasitology* 1972;64: 461–477

Owen J,M., "Liver fluke infection in horses and ponies," *Equine Vet J.* 1977 Jan;9(1):29-31.

Pandey VS. "Epidemiological observations on lungworm, *Dictyocaulus arnfieldi*, in donkeys from Morocco." *J Helminthol* (*Journal of Helminthology*) 1980

Paul JW. "Equine larval cyathostomosis." *Comp Cont Edu Pract Vet* 1998; 20: 509-513.

Payne, P.A., Carter, G.R., (Eds.).In *A Concise Guide to the Microbial and Parasitic Diseases of Horses*, Carter G.R., Payne P.A. and Davis E. International Veterinary Information Service, Ithaca NY (www.ivis.org), Last updated: 30-Nov-2007; A4703.1107

Pearson, W., "Ethnoveterinary Medicine: The Science of Botanicals in Equine Health and Disease," *Proceedings of the 2nd European Equine Health & Nutrition Congress*, (2003) Lelystad, The Netherlands, 31-40.

Pearson, W, Boermans, HJ, Bettger, WJ, McBride, BW, Lindinger, MI, 2004. "Safety assessment of freeze-dried garlic (Allium sativum) in horses: Heinz body anemia associated with maximum voluntary intake," *Am. J. Vet.* In Press.

Pearson, W., Boermans H.J., Betteger W.J., McBride B.W, Lindinger M.I., "Association of maximum voluntary dietary intake of freeze-dried garlic with Heinz body anemia in horses," *American Journal of Veterinary Research*, March 2005, Vol. 66, No. 3, 457-465.

Peregrine A, "Deworming programs for horses: are we doing more harm than good?" *As Presented in the Rounds of Department of Large Animal Clinical Sciences Western College of Veterinary Medicine*, June/July 2005, Vol. 5, Issue 6.

Peregrine A, McEwen B, Lusis P, *et. al.*, "Larval cyathostomiasis in horses: a new disease in Ontario?" *Animal Health Laboratory Newsletter*, University of Guelph 2002;6:22.

Proudman, CJ, French NP, Trees, AJ, "Tapeworm infection is a significant risk factor for spasmodic colic and ileal impaction colic in the horse," *Equine Vet J.* 1998; 30:194-199.

Purdy S.R., "Herd Health for Miniature Donkeys," In: *Veterinary Care of Donkeys*, Matthews N.S. and Taylor T.S. (Eds.). International Veterinary Information Service, Ithaca NY (www.ivis.org), Last updated: 1-Apr-2005; A2921.0405

Reid SWJ, Mair TS, Hillyer MH, Love S. "Epidemiological risk factors associated with a diagnosis of clinical cyathostomiasis in the horse." *Equine Vet J* (*Equine Veterinary Journal*) 1995; 27: 127-130.

Reinhart, K.M., Craig I Coleman, Colleen Teevan, Payal Vachhani, C Michael White, "Effects of Garlic on Blood Pressure in Patients With and Without Systolic Hypertension: A Meta-Analysis," *The Annals of Pharmacotherapy*, (2008) Vol. 42, No. 12, pp. 1766-1771.

Reinemeyer R, Henton JE. "Observations on equine strongyle control in southern temperate USA." *Equine Vet J* 1987;19:505–508.

Reinemeyer C.R., Douglas E. Hutchens, Wm. P. Eckblad, Alan A. Marchiondo and Jack I. Shugart "Dose-confirmation studies of the cestocidal activity of pyrantel pamoate paste in horses," *Veterinary Parasitology* Vol. 138, Issues 3-4, 15 June 2006.

Reinemeyer C.R., "Controlling Strongyle Parasites of Horses: A Mandate for Change," *Proceedings of the 55th Annual Convention of the American Association of Equine Practitioners*, 2009.

Reitsma, J.F. "The treatment of a lung worm infection in ponies with albendazole (Valbazen)." *Tijdschr Diergeneeskd* 1983; 108:569-571.

Rode B, Jorgensen RJ. "Baermannization of Dictyocaulus spp. from faeces of cattle, sheep and donkeys." *Vet Parasitol* 1989; 30:205-211.

Rolfe PF, Dawson KL, Holm-Martin M. "Efficacy of moxidectin and other anthelmintics against small strongyles in horses." *Aust Vet J* 1998;76:332–334.

Rose MA, Round MC, Beveridge WIB. "Influenza in horses and donkeys in Britain." *Vet Rec.* 1970; 86:768-769.

Round, M.C., "Lungworm infection (*Dictyocaulus arnfieldi*) of horses and donkeys." *Vet Rec* 1976; 99:393-395.

Round MC. *A study of the natural history of lungworm infection of equidae*. PhD Thesis, University of Cambridge, 1972.

Rupasinghe D, Ogbourne CP. "Laboratory studies on the effect of temperature on the development of the free-living stages of some strongylid nematodes of the horse." ZEITSCHRIFT FUR PFLANZENERNAHRUNG UND BODENKUNDE, 1978; 55:249–253.

Samson-Himmelstjerna von G, Fritzen B, Demeler J, Schurmann S, Rohn K, Schnieder T, Epe C, "Cases of reduced cyathostomin egg reappearance period and failure of Parascaris equorum egg count reduction following ivermectin treatment as well as survey on pyrantel efficacy on German horse farms." *Vet. Parasitol.* 2007

Satrija, F, "Anthelmintic activity of Indian mulberry fruit against Haemonchus contortus in sheep," *17th International Conference of WAAVP Copenhagen-Denmark* (f.5.02), 1999.

Satrija, F., Retnani, E.B., Ridwan, Y. and Tiuria, R., "Potential use of herbal anthelmintics as alternative antiparasitic drugs for small holder farms in developing countries," *Livestock Community and Environment. Proceedings of the 10th Conference of the Association of Institutions for Tropical Veterinary Medicine*, 2001, Copenhagen, Denmark.

Satrija, F., Nansen, P., Bjørn, H., Murtini, S. and He, S., "Effect of papaya latex (Carica papaya) against Ascaris suum in naturally infected pigs," *Journal of Helminthology*, 1994, 68: 343-346.

Satrija, F., P. Nansen, S. Murtini and He, S., "Anthelmintic activity of papaya latex against patent Heligmosomoides polygyrus infections in mice," *Journal of Ethnopharmacology*, (1995) 48: 161-164.

Schougaard H, Nielsen MK. "Apparent ivermectin resistance of Parascaris equorum in Danish foals." *Vet Rec* 2007;160:439–440.

Slocombe, J., De Gannes, R., "Effectiveness of moxidectin for benzimidazole and pyrantel resistant cyathostomes in horses," *Proceedings, 43rd Annual Meeting of the American Association of Veterinary Parasitologists* 1998

Slocombe, J., M. Lake, "Efficacy of Daily Pyrantel Tartrate (Strongid C) against Strongyles in Ponies on Pasture," *Journal of Equine Veterinary Science*, Volume 27, Issue 10, 439-445.

Slocombe JOD, de Gannes RVG, Lake MC. "Macrocyclic lactone-resistant Parascaris equorum on stud farms in Canada and effectiveness of fenbendazole and pyrantel pamoate." *Vet Parasitol* 2007;145:371–376.

Sollmann, T., "Anthelmintics: Their Efficiency as Tested on Earthworms," *Journal of Pharmacology And Experimental Therapeutics*, Vol. 12, Issue 3, 129-170, 1918.

Spears, J.W., E. B. Kegley, L. A. Mullis, "Bioavailability of copper from tribasic copper chloride and copper sulfate in growing cattle," *Animal Feed Science and Technology*, Volume 116, Issues 1-2, 1 September 2004, 1-13.

Stoneham S, Coles GC, "Ivermectin resistance in Parascaris equorum," Vet.Rec. 2006

Swiderski CE. "Equine parasitic disease". In: Smith B, ed. *Large animal internal medicine*, 4th ed. St. Louis: Mosby Inc., 2008.

Swiderski, C.E. and French, D.D., "Paradigms for Parasite Control in Adult Horse Populations: A Review." *54th Annual Convention of the American Association of Equine Practitioners* - AAEP, 2008 - San Diego, CA, USA.

Tarigo-Martinie, J.L., Wyatt, A.R., Kaplan, R.M. "Prevalence, clinical implications of anthelmintic resistance in cyathostomes of horses," *J Am Vet Med Assoc* 2001; 218, 1957-1960.

Thiemann A. K. and N. J. Bell, "The Peculiarities of Donkey Respiratory Disease." In: *Equine Respiratory Diseases*, Lekeux P. (Ed.) International Veterinary Information Service, Ithaca NY (www.ivis.org), 2001; B0330.1101 (Last Updated: 14-Nov-2001)

Trawford A.F. and Burden F. "Ivermectin resistance in cyathostomes in four donkeys herds at the Donkey Sanctuary, UK." *Worldwide Association for the Advancement of Veterinary Parasitology*, Calgary, 2009.

Turnlund, J.R., King JC, Gong B, Keyes WR, Michel MC, "A stable isotope study of copper absorption in young men: effect of phytate and a-cellulose," *Am J Clin Nutr* 1985;42:18–23.

Tyler, S.T., "The behavioural and social organisation of the New Forest pony," *Animal Behaviour Monographs* 5 (1972):96.

Uhlinger C, Kristula M. "Effects of alternation of drug classes on the development of oxibendazole resistance in a herd of horses." *J Am Vet Med* Assoc 1992;201:51–55.

Underwood, E. J., *Trace Elements in Human and Animal Nutrition*, (4th Ed.). Academic Press, 1977, New York.

Urch DL, Allen WR. "Studies on fenbendazole for treating lung and intestinal parasites in horses and donkeys." *Equine Vet J* 1980; 12:74-77.

Valle, E, Padalino, B, "Garlic Effects In the Horse; A Clinical Report," *Società Italiana Veterinari per Equini* - SIVE - XII *Congresso Multisala*, Bologna, Italy 2006.

Van Doorn DCK, Lems S, Weteling A, Ploeger HW, Eysker M, "Resistance of Parascaris equorum against ivermectin due to frequent anthelmintic treatment of foals in the Netherlands," *20th International Conference of the WAAVP*, Gent, 2007

Van Doorn DCK, and Harm W. Ploeger, "Worming horses the rational way " *European Veterinary Conference* Voorjaarsdagen Amsterdam, Netherlands 2008

Valero MA, S Mas-Coma, "Comparative infectivity of Fasciola hepatica metacercariae from isolates of the main and secondary reservoir animal host species in the Bolivian Altiplano high human endemic region," *Folia Parasitologica* 47, 2000, 17-22.

van Krimpen, M.M., G.P. Binnendijk, F. Borgsteede, C. Gaasenbeek, "In vivo testing of alternatives for conventional treatment of Ascaris suum in pigs," *Animal Sciences Group van Wageningen UR*, Rapport 82, November 2007, 17-21.

von Samson-Himmelstjerna G, Fritzen B, Demeler J, *et al*. "Cases of reduced cyathostomin egg-reappearance period and failure of Parascaris equorum egg count reduction following ivermectin treatment as well as survey on pyrantel efficacy on German horse farms." *Vet Parasitol* 2007

Ward, J.D., J. W. Spears 1, and E. B. Kegley, "Bioavailability of Copper Proteinate and Copper Carbonate Relative to Copper Sulfate in Cattle," *J Dairy Sci.* (1996) Jan;79 (1):127-32.

Webb R. "Epidemiological factors contributing to a high incidence of anthelmintic resistance in field populations in Haemonchus contortus." In: *Proceedings of the 2nd International Symposium on Veterinary Epidemiology and Economics* 1980;220–224.

Wilson, P.K. – 2005 Churchill Fellow, "Improving the Selection of Foreign Dung Beetle Species and Enhancing their Populations in Australia by Comparing the Effects of Grazing Activities in Natural and Transformed South African Environments," *The Winston Churchill Memorial Trust of Australia*, at http://www.dungbeetles.com.au/files/ChurchillTrustFinal.pdf

Winther, K., Kharazmi, A., "A powder prepared from seeds and shells of a subtype of rose-hip Rosa canina reduces pain in patients with osteoarthritis of the hand - a double-blind, placebo-controlled, randomized study," *Proceedings of the 9th World Congress OARSI*, Chicago, Dec. 04.

Yang, Qing, Qiuhui Hub, Osamu Yamatoc, Keun-Woo Leed, Yoshimitsu Maedec, Teruhiko Yoshiharaa, "Organosulphur Compounds from Garlic (Allium sativum) Oxidizing Canine Erythrocytes," *Z. Naturforsch.* 58c, 408Ð412 (2003).

9260647R0

Made in the USA
Lexington, KY
14 April 2011